Leo A. Gordon, MD

Cut to the Chase

100 Matrix Pearls for Doctors

tfm Publishing Limited
Castle Hill Barns
Harley
Nr Shrewsbury
SY5 6LX
UK
Tel: +44 (0)1952 510061; Fax: +44 (0)1952 510192
E-mail: nikki@tfmpublishing.com; Web site: www.tfmpublishing.com

Design: Nikki Bramhill
Typesetting: Nikki Bramhill
Front cover image: © 1999 Image 100 Ltd.

First Edition: August 2006
ISBN 1 903378 49 4

Printed by Gutenberg Press Ltd., Gudja Road, Tarxien, PLA 19, Malta.
Tel: +356 21897037; Fax: +356 21800069.

Contents

Preface

In the 1975 Woody Allen movie, *Love and Death*, two beleagured Russian soldiers are walking across the carnage and devastation of an 18th century battlefield. One of the characters, seeking a cosmic explanation for his situation, looks plaintively at Boris Grushenko (the Woody Allen character) and says: "Oh! God is testing us." Boris replies: "If he's gonna test us, why doesn't he give us a written?"

As a second year surgical resident, I knew exactly what Mr. Allen had in mind by this response. The disparity between the theoretical and the practical was just as marked for me as a surgical resident, as it was for the two soldiers in the film. I was in the midst of the very practical test that is a surgical education. I was armed with only the theoretical principles of surgery. I was prepared for the written exam. But the process of surgical education forced me to live in the world of the practical exam. I wished on many nights that I was participating in a written exam, rather than the real-life situations with which I was forced to deal.

The disparity between the theoretical and the real is a constant theme in all aspects of education. Nowhere is the gulf between the classroom and the real world more obvious than in the field of surgical education. The very nature of surgery, with its direct confrontation of disease, makes it so. Unlike other areas of medicine, one cannot function in surgery in a "written" mode.

The practical nature of surgery dictates that this gulf between the written and the practical be bridged. It is the obligation of medical educators to prepare the resident for the practical examination - the daily life of clinical medicine.

A surgical education program must fulfill that obligation. It must place the surgical resident in "battlefield" situations and teach him how to respond. Day after day, year after year with supervision and review, the new recruit becomes an experienced warrior - an educated surgeon.

There are, however, current deficiencies in this process. The two soldiers in *Love and Death* are less concerned with the general's battle plans than they are with a warm meal and a pair of dry socks! The generals live in a world of strategic theory and philosophy. The foot soldier lives in the trenches. The education designed by the surgical generals needs to be enhanced by a practical guide for daily surgical life. That brief cinematic exchange thirty years ago in a Boston movie theater planted the seed for many of these Matrix Lessons. I needed to know how to get an angiogram at midnight. I did not need to know the effects of 2,3, diethyl etc. I needed to know how to speak to families. I did not need to know that Professor Charnley always uses albumin.

I realized at that time that there are two sets of parallel surgical principles.

One set teaches:

- If the end-diastolic pressure exceeds 43 cm sq per kg of body weight, then the dose of the alpha adnergic stimulant should be ....
- Divide the areas of the neck into zones I, II, and III ...
- Never let the sun rise or set on a small bowel obstruction ...

These lessons are important. They are discussed year after year by various tenured professors of surgery. However, these laws govern a different type of surgical existence - the existence of theory and postulate; the life of the faculty lounge, the research building and the retreat.

Surgeons need more than the laws governing the theoretical aspects of surgical existence. Most surgeons do not live in the faculty lounge. They live in the emergency room or the ward, often in the middle of the night.

I came to realize that another set of equally important lessons exists.

This set of lessons teaches:

- If the gynecologist says it is adnexal, it is never adnexal.
- Never discuss the asymptomatic carotid bruit.
- Never let the patient near an interventional radiologist on a Friday.

These are the practical lessons of the emergency room, the ward and the operating theater. These are the lessons that govern day-to-day practical surgical existence. Such practical lessons existed only as some great oral surgical tradition handed down from resident to resident.

An oral surgical culture had developed which had never recorded the most practical information governing its daily life. Ironically, these lessons were discussed weekly at the surgical morbidity and mortality conference. But the conference consistently failed its participants. There was never a method of distilling all of the practical knowledge discussed at this essential weekly conclave.

I decided to correct that by developing the *M + M Matrix Program* and by fostering the Matrix concept. These Matrix Lessons are practical lessons learned at the Matrix Conference.

I offer these Matrix Lessons as a canon for the working physician.

Leo A. Gordon, MD
Los Angeles, California

Introduction

I recently completed twenty-six years of surgical practice at a major metropolitan medical center with an international reputation and easy freeway access to recreational areas.

I sat in our hospital coffee shop in a reflective mood sipping my coffee. The new chief resident came over to chat. This is how it is on the American West Coast - "chatting" with the attending surgeon. It was a far different state of affairs in the mid-nineteen seventies on the East Coast. The closest thing to a "chat" I ever had with any surgical attending was a perfunctory bow in the hallway - but that is for another book.

That resident and I discussed many things about the upcoming year. We focused on what he had learned in the past four years and how he was about to apply it to this year. For this would be "his" year - the crowning achievement of four years of hard work - a year of refinement of skills and of honing that razor-sharp surgical mind.

What advice could I give him? What could I share with him? (The West Coast is also big on "sharing." As near as I can figure it "sharing" is just like "chatting," only longer).

I began listing several important pieces of advice for him. It struck me that all of the advice was rather practical, maybe even mundane. The advice involved the day-to-day functioning of a busy surgical service and practice. We talked less about the physiology of septic shock than about the machinations of the radiology department. We spoke briefly about the technical aspects of pancreatic resections, but endlessly about diagnostic restraint. I mentioned some issues of breast disease. I also discussed the absolute futility of trying to control the surgical day.

Essentially, we discussed the practical laws of daily surgical life as opposed to the theoretical and technical aspects of that life. As the conversation progressed, I started to list these practical lessons I had learned over the course of my own career.

It became clear to me that most of this practical knowledge had been analyzed during discussions at our morbidity and mortality conference. But our conference, as with such conferences throughout the country had no mechanism for recording, memorializing and distributing this valuable information - information one cannot find in standard surgical texts.

The M & M Matrix Program was born.*

Since that discussion, our morbidity and mortality conference has been reconfigured, redefined and re-invented via the M+M Matrix. The Matrix concept generates a weekly error and complication-reducing curriculum from the points made at the traditional surgical morbidity and mortality conference. The lessons of the morbidity and mortality conference became lessons in patient safety.

Such a patient safety effort had never been done in this manner in the history of organized surgical education. The public demands patient safety. Surgical educators are obligated to create a culture of patient safety at the inception of surgical education. At its best the surgical morbidity and mortality conference is a patient safety conference. At worst it is a useless exercise in shame and blame that has probably

* Gordon LA. Can Cedars-Sinai's M+M Matrix Save Surgical Education? *Bulletin of the American College of Surgeons* 2004; 89(6): 16-20.

driven thousands of eager fourth year students away from this great discipline.

To change the culture of a conference, the first place to start is with its name. There should be no more morbidity and mortality conferences. There should only be Matrix Conferences - conferences that take the lessons of an error or a complication and construct a curriculum of safety around them. These are the lessons that comprise this book.

Except for Matrix Lesson #1, the lessons in this book are not listed in any particular order of importance or preference. The lessons mirror the surgical day - sporadic, uneven, random and impossible to organize. Although most of the Matrix Lessons are surgically oriented, they have applicability to all areas of medicine.

The lessons discussed govern the nuts and bolts of medical practice. They have been tested and are quite functional. True to surgical form, they are personal and opinionated.

Read these Matrix Lessons. Use them as you see fit. Above all, enjoy them!

Leo A. Gordon, MD
Los Angeles, California

What is a Matrix Lesson?

A Matrix Lesson is an essential medical error and complication-reducing point, an experienced medical observation or a trenchant medical insight reduced to a concise lesson statement

To understand these Matrix Lessons, the reader must be familiar with the traditional surgical morbidity and mortality conference. This conference is a weekly meeting held in many hospitals. At this meeting the errors and complications of the previous week are discussed. A resident (a postgraduate physician) presents the case to the audience. The floor is then open for comments.

The goal of this conference is to analyze error and complication and, in so doing, to plant a seed of patient-safety consciousness in all of those who attend.

The traditional morbidity and mortality conference has failed its mission. The error and complication-reducing lessons so vital to the safe practice of medicine are often lost in a mish-mash of prejudice, myth and medical anecdote. In many quarters of American medicine, this time-honored weekly assemblage has degenerated into a useless game of shame and blame.

The goal of the morbidity and mortality conference has always been to teach error and complication-reducing lessons. Unfortunately, the conference has come to resemble an aboriginal tribe that never invented a written language. The best minds of the hospital, whetted by spirited debate and passion, often delivered concrete and valuable lessons for physicians - lessons that would help them prevent errors and avoid complications. But no-one ever recorded those lessons for the future.

In an attempt to correct these deficiencies, some progressive departments of surgery have transformed the morbidity and mortality conference into a Matrix Conference.

A Matrix Conference is a moderated discussion of a reported complication or medical error. This discussion seeks to define the essential error and complication-reducing points of the presentation. The moderator records them and then distributes them. These essential principles become Matrix Lessons.

Many Matrix Lessons are learned from the practice of medicine outside of the conference. They all intertwine along the highways and byways of the medical center - the patient's room, the hospital corridors, the operating rooms, the doctors' lounge, the residents' lounge and the doctors' offices.

A philosopher once said: "Experience is a hard teacher because she gives the test first, the lesson afterwards." The one hundred lessons that follow are those lessons learned from thirty years' attendance at the morbidity and mortality conference. They are also the lessons learned from one hundred tests administered by a hard teacher - the clinical practice of medicine.

Acknowledgements

Many people played a role in the formulation of these Matrix Lessons. The lessons were written from the daily give-and-take at all levels of a medical center. Most of the lessons arose from the Matrix Conference discussions. Many of them were generated from an insightful e-mail, a hallway comment or a telephone call from a colleague.

I found one particular proving ground quite helpful in formulating and refining the lessons. I eat lunch with a group of disparate physicians. Internists, surgeons, radiologists, and other specialists gravitate to a round table in our coffee shop. These physicians bring to this table the length and breadth of the American medical experience. The discussions arising from these lunchtime debates and diatribes helped me to formulate many of the lessons.

Several individuals were most helpful.

I will forever be indebted to Dr. Achilles Demetriou, former Chief of Surgery at the Cedars-Sinai Medical Center. Dr. Demetriou is a great supporter of the Matrix concept. It was he who allowed me to begin the Matrix Program in the Department that he chaired. His support was vital to the inception of the Program and has been a vital force in allowing the concept to spread throughout the surgical world.

I must acknowledge the contributions of Dr. David Cossman (Vascular Surgery). His attempts to explain the asymptomatic carotid bruit led to the formulation of one of the more amusing lessons (Matrix Lesson #43) in this book. His guidance regarding the syntax and format of this book was most helpful. Dr. Cossman is the apotheosis of the clinical surgeon - that rare combination of clinical insight, technical brilliance and medical practicality.

Dr. Allan Silberman, fellow resident, colleague and friend has played a great role in the formulation of these lessons. We discovered surgery together. In the illogical world of academia, we had to forge a practical and enjoyable existence. He helped with both. His support and encouragement are appreciated. Dr. Silberman is the only true professor of surgery I have ever met. He is the only "contributor" to this effort who so influenced the lesson of the Matrix (Matrix Lesson #10) that the lesson became eponymous.

I thank Dr. Leon Morgenstern, Emeritus Director of Surgery at the Cedars-Sinai Medical Center for his guidance and editorial stewardship. Dr. Morgenstern's dedication and allegiance to the core principles of medical education have helped more physicians and patients than he could ever imagine.

Now to the members of the Medical House and Senate who argued these lessons and made the ideas in the book come alive: Dr. Michael Van-Scoy Mosher (oncology/hematology), Dr. Carol Hyman (pediatric hematology), Drs. Stuart Holden and Dudley Danoff (urology), Dr. Frank Moser, Dr. Marcel Maya and Dr. James Tourje (radiology), Dr. Martin Cooper (neurosurgery), and Dr. Jeffrey Helfenstein, Dr. Mark Erman, Dr. Jeffrey Caren (cardiology/internal medicine), Dr. Julian Gold and Dr. Thomas Webb (anesthesiology), Dr. Andrew Wachtel (pulmonology), Dr. Franklin Strauss (nephrology), Dr. Robert Gerber (dentist), Dr. Millard Zisser (dermatology), Dr. Larry Richman and Dr. Dan Rovner (neurology) - each through his own unique approach to medical practice contributed a particular perspective on the practical lessons of clinical medicine. More appreciated than their contributions to this book is their valued friendship.

Luis in Plant Operations provided many insights into the construction of surgeons' lounges.

Many of the Matrix Lessons are resident-oriented. Surgical residents helped me immensely as they sought my counsel and my limited wisdom. I thank them for the privilege of showing them the light of insight along the dark and serpiginous path of a surgical education.

Since surgical residents have trouble paying attention and can only understand nuggets of intelligence, I disciplined myself to speak to them in lesson-like fashion. An elegantly stated, tightly worded lesson in surgery has more impact on a resident than a lengthy diatribe or scholarly discourse. The need by the resident for a compact statement helped me to streamline many of my thoughts into lesson-like guidelines.

I owe a special debt to the many surgical nurses who have cared for my patients over the years. Their dedication and insight are appreciated. Their activities formed the basis for many of the lessons.

The astute reader may say after reading through this text, "Hey! I've heard it all before!" or "God, I heard that when I was a resident!" Many of the lessons are simply part of surgical lore - that great body of verbal knowledge that is passed down from year to year. I have made every effort to search for the author of each to give full credit.

If anyone can accurately provide me with the first person to state the idea contained in one of the lessons, please contact me and credit will be given in future editions.

Cut to the Chase came to life due in great part to the editorial assistance, guidance and brilliant layout expertise of Ms. Nikki Bramhill and the staff at tfm publishing. Their trans-Atlantic patience, sense of humor and insight into the medical mind represent a special place in medical publishing.

I owe the greatest debt to the thousands of surgical patients with whom I have come in contact. These people have been plucked from their otherwise orderly existence and have been hurled headlong into the maelstrom of a surgical day. They were instantaneously taken out of their world - comfortable and familiar - and were thrust into the world of the clinical physician - hectic, emergent and often chaotic. They allowed me to be their guide through that world. For that I am most grateful.

Leo A. Gordon, MD
Los Angeles, California

Author biography

Leo A. Gordon MD, is one of America's leading medical educators. His reconfiguration of the traditional morbidity and mortality (audit) conference has attracted international attention. His lectures and seminars on transforming this essential conference into a vibrant patient safety program have played a major role in the patient safety movement.

Born in New England, schooled in the Midwest, Dr. Gordon received his surgical education in Boston. He has practiced general surgery in Los Angeles for over twenty-six years.

Dr. Gordon is the author of *Gordon's Guide to the Surgical Morbidity and Mortality Conference,* described by the *Journal of the American Medical Association* as a "... cult classic to be."

Dr. Gordon serves on the editorial board and is a frequent contributor to *General Surgery News,* America's most widely read surgical news monthly.

He is the originator of the M+M Matrix - an error and complication-reducing medical curriculum generated from the morbidity and mortality conference.

Est igitur haec non scripta sed nata lex; quam nun dedicimus accepimus, legimus, verum ex natura ipsa arripuimus, hausimus, expressiumu; as quam non docti, sed facti, non instituti sed imbuti sumus.

This, therefore, is a law not found in books, but written on the fleshy tablets of the heart, which we have not learned from man, received or read, but which we have caught up from nature herself, sucked in and imbibed; the knowledge of which we were not taught, but for which we were made; we received it not by education, but by intuition.

Cicero

For

Jack and Minna

Ward and Jean

Jan, Ari and Jason

Judy and Jerry

19215

Matrix Lesson 1

The Matrix Conference is the most important hour of the surgical week

Nihil est tam insigne, nec tam ad
diurnitatem memoriae stabile, quam id,
in quo aliquid offenderis.
Cicero De Oratore, I, 129

Nothing stands out so conspicuously,
or remains so firmly fixed in our
memory, as something in which we
have blundered.

Before the Institute of Medicine Report; before the medical liability crisis; before investigative news teams with stylized unemployed English majors schlepping around town in video vans; before all of this, there was the surgical morbidity and mortality conference.

This conference - a weekly meeting to discuss medical errors and complications - is the single greatest patient safety mechanism ever conceived. Unfortunately, full-term delivery never followed this brilliant conception.

Under the aegis of some of the greatest names in American surgery, the surgical morbidity and mortality conference devolved into a useless shame and blame political-surgical game. At the center of this game, like a chit on a gameboard, was a surgical chief resident.

Fortunately for American medicine, the morbidity and mortality conference has been reconfigured via an innovative concept called the *M+M Matrix* or *Matrix Conference*. A morbidity and mortality conference becomes a Matrix Conference by generating a patient safety curriculum from the points made during these discussions.

Anyone can analyze a medical success. But it takes intelligence and a concern for the advancement of your own development to analyze a medical failure.

The weekly Matrix Conference analyzes medical failure. Much can be learned from those analyses at every level of the surgical food chain - from the chief of surgery to the surgical intern.

A well-run, well-supported and well-attended Matrix Conference is the single greatest source of surgical education. This conference is the last bastion of dispassionate medical debate. It is a special event when a surgeon bears his surgical soul to his colleagues. There is nothing like it in all of medicine.

The interplay at the Matrix Conference is a fascinating study. The dynamic between the presenting resident and the audience, the various components of that audience and how they interact against a framework of surgical practice and principle make for a lively and educational meeting.

Whether you are an intern or a seasoned attending, a well-run Matrix Conference is the greatest adjunct to one's ongoing education.

This conference sets the surgical ship of state on the proper course. Analyzing errors of judgment, technique and diagnosis exposes surgical ignorance in a group setting. It is a powerful tool.

There is a varying commitment to this meeting from institution to institution. I would hope that this most rigorous of meetings will always be a central part of any division of surgery.

"Anyone can analyze a medical success. But it takes intelligence and a concern for the advancement of your own development to analyze a medical failure."

The key to a successful meeting relies on several factors:

- The resident must be prepared for it.
- Attendance for surgeons whose patients have suffered the complication should be mandatory.
- The co-ordinator of the meeting must be prepared and committed to the meeting as a valuable educational tool for the entire division of surgery.
- The division of surgery itself must support the meeting with appropriate secretarial and audio-visual staff.
- The division must view the meeting as infinitely more important than the nurse-liaison, emeritus parking or physician well-being committee meetings.

Combining these five elements will enhance attendance and will give value to the discussions at the Matrix Conference.

Fortunately for the discipline of surgery, the definitive guide to this most important hour has been written.* All one has to do is plug *Gordon's Guide* into your favorite search engine, get out the plastic and press "submit."

* See *The Journal of the American Medical Association* 1995: 273(1): 86-7.

Matrix Lesson 2

A referral to a surgical office

never generates a surgical case

No surgical referral, in the elective office setting, ever generates a bona fide surgical case. To the uninitiated this may seem like a strange statement. An example will make this clear.

Here is a recent office visit log*:

1. Jones, Alan - gastric lesion.
2. Carter, Sylvia - breast cancer.
3. Miles, Warren - ventral hernia.
4. Wilson, Mary - rectal tumor.

At first glance, this office list is a working surgeon's dream. The cases seem interesting, and of more significance, actually appear to be surgical cases. Any

* These are not the real names of the patients in order to protect their identity.

surgeon worth his weight in utilization review notices is envisioning the following week's work: gastrectomy, mastectomy, repair of body wall hernia, excision of rectal lesion.

His mind is agog with the many ways his expertise will be challenged. Where is the gastric lesion? Will I need to do a total gastrectomy? What type of reconstruction will I use? The patient with breast cancer - is she a candidate for sentinel node excision? Has she explored options? The patient with the ventral hernia - will I need a synthetic reconstruction of the body wall? The man with the rectal lesion - is he elderly? Should I offer transanal excision? Will I be able to do a low anterior resection?

"No surgical referral, in the elective office setting, ever generates a bona fide surgical case."

Such an office list gets the surgical juices flowing. It suffuses the surgeon with a sense of worth and actually makes him look forward to going to his office - an unusual feeling for most surgeons who would rather be in the operating room or in the surgeons' lounge.

But let us see how this surgical dream list played out:

1. The gastric lesion was nothing more than a prominent rugal fold, over-read by a radiologist. A subsequent endoscopy proved this.

2. The breast cancer patient was new to town. She had undergone a mastectomy twenty years ago and was here to establish surgical follow-up care.

3. The ventral hernia was a *diastasis recti* inappropriately referred by the internist.

4. The rectal lesion was an asymptomatic skin tag.

All of this was relatively good news for the patients. But the working surgeon, glad as he is for the good fortune of his patients, is somewhat disappointed. The week's challenges and week's work have evaporated.

Hopes dashed, frustration mounting, the surgeon leaves his office for the hospital, the ward or the emergency room, where surgical referrals actually materialize into surgical cases.

Matrix Lesson 3

Any case presented as: "See the patient when you can at your convenience" is a four-plus-flat-out surgical emergency with a mortality of 98% and should be seen immediately

"Obverse of Law #3: any case presented as: 'See the patient immediately. He needs surgery now!' will never need surgery."

The nonchalance of the referral process is sneaky. There is an inverse relationship with the urgency of the consult request as outlined above. The "see it when you can" case has been festering under the sheets for at least two days. The leisurely after-office evening consult is usually a neglected colon obstruction that will land you in the operating theater at about midnight. The "see it now" case is seldom urgent.

Who can explain this? Is it that our colleagues do not recognize surgical disease? Is it abject ignorance? For some reason, urgency is a surgical trait.

After the explosion of wonder drugs and sophisticated imaging techniques, most of the medical world fell in love with the concept and theory of disease. Working surgeons, on the other hand, look at a clinical problem and think: what am I missing that can kill this guy?

More importantly, surgeon's think anatomically - the only physicians who still think in this manner. Only the working surgeons of the world held on to functional anatomic principles - the principles at work in surgical disease. Surgeons constantly think anatomically. The distended abdomen is not just distension; it is intestinal necrosis and death. The abdominal pain is not just abdominal pain; it is a dead gallbladder or a ruptured appendix with sepsis. Our anatomic view of the world lends urgency to every problem and instills in the surgical consultant a desire to define and cure that problem.

To an increasingly noticeable degree, this approach is lacking in other specialties. When another physician sees distension all he thinks about is the amorphous concept of distension. This fuzzy theoretical approach lessens the immediacy of treatment. This colors the tone of the request to the surgeon.

Occasionally, these managing physicians may regard a clinical situation as emergent. They are usually wrong. I sat next to Billy Garfield in the sixth grade. For the eight years of mathematics, Billy was always two integers away from the correct answer. Billy tried to add, subtract, multiply and divide. Despite extra sessions, tutoring and coaching, he would always be off by about two. Billy's disciples grew up to be the guys who call you urgently to see a patient who, engrossed in Monday night football says as you enter the room: "Gosh, Doc, you're working late tonight!"

Having explained now how to respond to urgent and leisurely consults, we will concentrate on the delicate art of calling the physician back and explaining to him your thoughts. Self-control is important. Most of these conversations end with the referring physician saying: "Yes, that's just what I thought!"

Matrix Lesson 4

Never study an improving situation

Among the medical activities that fascinate me, none is more intriguing than the desire of many of my colleagues to study an improving situation.

Here is a patient who has gone through an operation. Perhaps there is a complication and a re-operation. Perhaps there has been a long and difficult recovery. Now, the patient is getting better. Slowly, incrementally, day by day, he looks better. He feels better. He actually is better by every parameter available to the surgical team, including that most ephemeral parameter - how he "looks" coming through the door. And yet, someone feels compelled to order a study. To prove, if you will, what one already knows.

Saul Richmond was just such a patient. Saul was seventy years old. He had been through two wars and had built a successful business. In the grand American tradition, he was all set to relax and enjoy. He sold his business, sold his house and was preparing for retirement. He had chronic ulcer disease. He had exhausted current medical treatment. He underwent a vagotomy and antrectomy. Postoperatively, he developed a well-controlled, low-output duodenal-cutaneous fistula. Two weeks after surgery, Saul was improving to the point of tolerating a regular diet.

"Never study an improving situation."

A member of the surgical team caring for Saul was an enterprising intern. Fresh from the professorial fistula lecture he decided to order a barium contrast study to "define the anatomy of the fistula." The intern later related at the morbidity and mortality conference that, according to the lecture, such anatomic definition was essential should the patient develop a problem in the future. The Professor had stressed this in his lecture. The surgical team, the intern reasoned, would then have a "map" of Mr. Richmond's fistula, allowing them to better care for him. The intern sent Saul to radiology for a "sinogram upper GI." The ward clerk, however, only transposed the "upper GI" part of the order. Saul was transported to radiology. There, he was offered the usual oil barrel of barium. Dutifully, he drank it. Saul vomited and aspirated the barium. He died of a respiratory arrest in the radiology suite.

Instead of being in his living room watching a Celtics game, Saul was buried at a veterans' cemetery in Boston. The intern was at the funeral at the command of the chief resident. This was back in the days when a chief resident had clout and influence. I suppose if that same chief resident were here today he would probably be hauled before the Physicians' Well Being Committee for being unduly harsh on his junior residents and certainly for not paying enough attention to the intern's psychosocial needs in a stress-filled non-nurturing environment.

Saul Richmond survived two wars and a depression, but he was not strong enough to survive the misguided curiosity of a surgical automaton who needed to "define the anatomy" by studying an improving situation.

Never study an improving situation.

Matrix Lesson 5

A patient cannot sleep through peritonitis

You can sleep through a nephrology lecture. You can sleep through the grand rounds topic "Does 2,3, diethyl pseudocholinesterase inhibit adrenal response in hypophysectomized Wistar rats?" You can sleep through resident evaluation sessions, and even the chief's Christmas party. But a human being cannot sleep through peritonitis.

The patient with peritonitis lies quietly in bed. The patient with peritonitis is ill. The patient with peritonitis does not want to move. The patient with peritonitis cannot sleep.

So it follows, then, that if you are called urgently to see a patient, and that patient is, in fact, sleeping, it is unlikely that that particular patient will require your surgical expertise at that point.

Residents and referring doctors often wonder why, when summoned to see a patient in the middle of the night, I will get to the threshold of the room, observe the patient, and then return home. I do this most frequently when called upon to rule out appendicitis.

"Observation is a dying art in this day of CT scans and MRIs. Nevertheless, in many situations it can be a useful adjunct to making early decisions."

I am not a sleep expert (to me, the answer to all sleep problems is Postum™), but I realized early in my career that a patient cannot sleep through the process of peritonitis.

Sleep is restful. Sleep is unencumbered by care. Sleep is the sweet refresher that ravels up the worried sleeve of care.* The face of the sleeping person is that of a relaxed person. It is extremely unlikely that a patient with peritonitis requiring surgery will be able to sleep through the ordeal.

Because of this insight, I instruct residents to remember the time-honored requirement of the surgeon to *observe the patient* prior to performing any exams. Observation is a dying art in this day of CT scans and MRIs. Nevertheless, in many situations it can be a useful adjunct to making early decisions.

If you observe the patient, and that patient is truly sleeping, let the patient sleep. When I am in this situation, I usually just leave a note: "See you in the morning. Did not want to wake you up. Regards, Dr. Gordon."

Then *I* go to sleep!

---

* This is not original with me.

Matrix Lesson 6

Those patients seen on rounds
do not need to be seen on rounds

"Obverse of Law #6. Those patients **not seen** on rounds have manifestations of an early surgical **complication** that could have been **detected** on **rounds**."

If something is round it is smooth, uninterrupted and ends where it began. Whoever named the morning and evening activities of surgeons must have been more of a mathematician and geometrician than a surgeon. Daily surgical rounds are fragmented, irregular, constantly interrupted and anything but smooth.

The more appropriate geometric term to describe such surgical activity would be "scattergram." "Dr. Flieber is making scattergrams" is more surgically accurate than "Dr. Flieber is making rounds."

The exigencies of the surgical day in a busy practice prevent the cautious and uninterrupted ritual the public thinks is rounds. Emergency phone calls, office pressures, surgical schedules, post-prandial gastrointestinal emergencies from cafeteria food - all conspire to make rounds a pressure-packed time challenge, rather than a Marcus Welby retrospective. For these reasons, patients sometimes are missed on these visits. Plans are then made to see these patients "later in the day."

Matrix Lesson #6 addresses the fact that those people who are seen do not need to be seen and those people who are missed, with great probability, will have an evolving problem which should have been seen and addressed. There is absolutely no way around this, since if you see the person who needs to be seen, magically, his problem will disappear.

Rounds are a grand tradition in surgery. Experienced surgeons and residents realize early in their careers that it is the nature of surgery to deliver the unexpected and the unanticipated. Lesson #6 addresses this in a clear and succinct fashion.

Of course, if *all* patients are seen on rounds, which actually happened in Cleveland on November 17th 1968, you can forget this Lesson.

Matrix Lesson 7

Never allow a patient near an interventional radiologist on a Friday afternoon, at night or during a weekend

Interventional radiologists are the current-day analogues of the early Paleolithic seeker-hunters. In Paleolithic days, these primitive types would stalk their prey. Then, using crude spears and poles, would impale their prey.

The dilemma at that point was simply, what to do with the prey. Since they had not yet discovered fire, freezer bags, means of transport, or the minimum daily requirement vitamin charts, they were perplexed as to what to do with that dead organism. It was the *hunt* that captivated them - not the kill. Standing there, they pondered and pondered. Then ... they left.

This anthropological-historical act is played out every Friday afternoon at major medical centers throughout the world. Instead of Bronze Age implements tied to wooden spears, the radiological Ur-hunter uses wire catheters and metallic needles.

"... schedule the **involvement** of an interventional **radiologist** ... at a time when the **patient** will have the **benefit** of a **team approach**."

To approach and capture his prey, he no longer relies on foot-prints, olfactory clues or droppings (although all of these are in evidence in any busy radiology department). He is guided by CAT scans, MRIs and ultrasounds. The techniques are different, but the hunting spirit is the same.

As tumors are biopsied, stents are placed, arteries are dilated and abscesses are drained, this anthropologic throwback culminates with the prey left behind. The hunter disappears into the mists of the evening weekend. The wounded prey must then rely on others for help.

Calling on the services of the radiological Ur-hunter requires sophisticated judgment by the managing surgeon. The best time to employ their services is early on a Monday morning. It should be made clear to the Head of the radiologic Ur-tribe that his involvement does not end with the placement of the spear. Rather, it begins with that act.

Experienced surgeons involve interventional radiologists in the management of their patients with the expressed understanding of four important facts:

- Placing a spear engenders certain responsibilities.
- Problems can arise from spear placement.
- One can minimize the more cumbersome aspects (midnight surgery, off-hour mobilization of operating room and nursing

personnel, etc.) of those problems by scheduling spear-placement at appropriate times when the hospital and the surgeons are at peak efficiency.

■ The responsibility for managing these problems, though resting primarily with the surgeon, is shared by the spear-placer.

Surgical patients and their surgeons are victims of the random nature of surgical pathology. Such pathology always strikes at the most inopportune time. Matrix Lesson #7 teaches us to schedule the involvement of an interventional radiologist, if the condition of the patient allows, at a time when the patient will have the benefit of a team approach should a problem arise.

Matrix Lesson 8

Last year's study, "reportedly normal," is *always* abnormal

Along with the general decline in enthusiasm and intelligence of surgical house officers has come a most loathsome tendency. That tendency is to accept, without question, the word-of-mouth results of an investigative test which could easily have been retrieved and verified.

Why is it we can get "The Best of Boxcar Willie" over-night delivered to our door, yet last month's CT scan is put on the same scale as the Holy Grail? The answer is simple: the resident or surgeon surrenders to the minimal difficulty presented by attempting to retrieve an old study.

We will accept the challenge of a necrotic splenic flexure. We revel in the dilemma of the adherent tumor. We bask in the glow of a neatly dissected tumor. Yet we cringe at the prospect of intellectually digging out the data. Why? Why do we rely on word of mouth when with minimal effort we can get to the source?

We should approach pre-operative data in the same way as we approach a surgical anatomic challenge. Show me that last year's X-ray was "normal." Get those slides that were read as "negative." If one is planning an operation and one is basing decisions and plans on that data, one should be reasonably confident that the data are reliable.

You will often find that the upper gastrointestinal study in Dallas was not normal; that the CT done last year in Cedar Rapids was not "essentially negative" and that the biopsy from Tampa, on review, was really quite revealing.

The impact this lesson has is greatest when the unsuspecting presenter at the Matrix Conference is called upon to review last year's "normal" study which some enterprising, though heartless attending, has taken the time to retrieve.

Outlining that six-centimeter lesion in the cecum in front of the entire division of surgery brings the philosophy of Matrix Lesson #8 home in a most instructive and unforgettable manner.

"If one is planning an operation and one is basing decisions and plans on that data, one should be reasonably confident that the data are reliable."

Matrix Lesson 9

The scrub nurse will discuss lunch relief
at the most critical juncture of the case

Splenic artery slipped away? Posterior row of the low anterior resection slithering into the depths of the pelvis? Fifth attempt at cannulation of the cystic duct during laparoscopic cholecystectomy about to take place? Tumor abutting the ureter at a critical stage of the dissection about to be approached? There is a 99% chance that at that most critical surgical moment; at that apex of surgical judgment the nurse will proclaim: "Sally - lunch relief!"

Two widely disparate areas are thus juxtaposed: a critical surgical move and the leisure of lunch. The inanity of this disparity converges within the surgeon's cortex resulting in what neuropsychologists call *spielkes*.

Why does the nutritional replenishment of the nursing service always intrude at the most critical juncture of an operation? Why, at the moment of the surgeon's greatest need to concentrate and focus must the image of lunch be invoked?

"The talent involved in announcing lunch relief in perfect co-ordination with difficult surgical moves is a pre-requisite for co-ordinating busy operating rooms."

Somewhere in the *Big Book of Nurse Rules* is the precept: discuss lunch relief only when the surgeon is in the middle of a critical surgical move! To understand this nursing rule, we must understand the dynamics of one Ms. Sylvia McArdle, civil war nurse.

Sylvia McArdle was attached to the Massachusetts Third Division. During the Battle of Antietam, she was arranging lunch relief during a critical time in the evacuation of the Third Haverhill Battalion. She corralled the nurses and led them to the lunch tent just as an incoming Confederate mortar shell hit the regiment, wiping out most of the soldiers. This event imprinted the importance of lunch relief onto the annals of nursing. It made lunch the top priority of the nursing day.

The Smithsonian has the original McArdle lunch relief schedule of April 3, 1862. It is a must-see for surgeons visiting Washington.

It is uncanny how nurses have preserved Ms. McArdle's legacy. The talent involved in announcing lunch relief in perfect co-ordination with difficult surgical moves is a pre-requisite for co-ordinating busy operating rooms. Just as the needle tip is coming into view from the depths of a moving abyss, just as the stapling device is being fired, culminating three hours of mid-rectal mobilization, just as the aortic suture line begins to resemble the Fountain of Trevi and just when your surgical focus is clear and your talents most needed, comes the shrill cry based on the one thing furthest from your mind and your own surgical needs: "Alice - did you get lunch relief?"

Matrix Lesson 10

Never forget Silberman's rule: he who refuses a colostomy, *always* gets a colostomy

"Corollary #1 of Silberman's rule: the colostomy he gets will be performed under urgent circumstances. Corollary #2 of Silberman's rule: the colostomy he gets will be permanent."

I have heard many reasons for avoiding the performance of a colostomy, the most specious of which is, simply: "The patient wanted to avoid a colostomy."

Other groaners are: "I wanted to save him a second operation." Or, my personal favorite: "The family did not want him to get one."

Last time I checked in most standard surgical texts, the wants and desires of the patient or his family really did not have much to do with the surgical judgment as to whether or not to perform a colostomy. There is a curious wind of fate that blows through the surgical ward (are you getting the enteric metaphor here?) whenever a patient influences a decision to perform a colostomy. That wind is the powerful blast of Silberman's rule.

"The surgeon must do what is surgically appropriate, not what the patient wishes."

The more a surgeon wants to avoid something, the more likely it becomes that that something will come his way. This is especially true for the patient and the surgeon who, *for the wrong reasons*, avoids the performance of a colostomy.

Which brings us to corollary #1 of Silberman's rule. Having made a decision based on non-surgical principles, the need for the indicated operation arises then in the urgent setting. Yes, the colostomy was avoided, but now it is needed, usually on a Sunday afternoon with a patient in septic shock from a pelvic abscess. The colostomy is created under the most urgent of circumstances.

Which leads us to corollary #2 of Silberman's rule. The colostomy so desperately avoided, so urgently created is now ..... permanent! It is permanent for medical and metaphysical reasons. The medical reasons are clear. The patient is critically ill and will be lucky if he survives. The future colostomy closure then represents a prohibitive surgical risk. These medical reasons are subordinate to the metaphysical reason for corollary #2 - the surgeon and the patient tempted the Surgical Fates.

Both realize it and are not anxious to tempt Fate again. The colostomy remains.

Colostomies are often necessary and reflect good surgical judgment as part of many surgical procedures. The lay impression of colostomies, their surgery and their maintenance is unfortunately stuck circa 1958. Low anterior resections, rectal excisions, inflammatory bowel disease, urgent obstructive or perforative cases - many situations arise when a colostomy may be necessary and life-saving. Thankfully, advances in surgical techniques and the advent of enterostomal nursing have made the care and maintenance of colostomies tolerable. Still, many patients will be reluctant to undergo such procedures, putting a bind on the surgeon. The surgeon must do what is surgically appropriate, not what the patient wishes.

Matrix Lesson #10 - Silberman's rule - is one of the most reliable rules in all of clinical medicine. It is based on surgical judgment and common sense. It is a mainstay of the surgeon's commitment to the principles of safe surgery.

Matrix Lesson 11

The incidence of small bowel obstruction increases during Passover

---

The recognition and treatment of small bowel obstruction is an essential component of clinical surgical practice. Surgery for this entity can be straightforward (the lysis of a single adhesive band) or quite complex (the "cement abdomen" concretized by desmoplastic adhesions throughout the abdomen). Complications of surgery for small bowel obstruction are a frequent topic at the Matrix Conference. One area deserves special attention.

Many great and storied surgical programs are based at Jewish affiliated hospitals or are located in parts of metropolitan areas with large Jewish populations. It is important for surgeons to be ethnically sensitive to certain ritual celebrations which may lead to surgical disease. One such celebration is the holiday of Passover.

A clear relationship between bowel obstructions and Passover has been commented on at many Matrix Conferences. While never assessed in a rigorous scientific manner, the correlation is clear.

Passover, marking the flight of the Jews from Egypt, is celebrated every Spring. As the story goes, Jewish slaves, in a hurry to leave Egypt did not have time to let their baking bread rise. In their haste, they hurried out of Egypt with unleavened cakes. These unleavened cakes are called *matzoh*. If you have never eaten matzoh, you have denied yourself one of the great culinary experiences available to human-kind. I prefer egg-matzoh, available at many stores. I slather it with margarine and strawberry jam and eat it all during Passover, which I think runs fourteen days.

I should point out as of this writing, that I am a healthy male, well hydrated with excellent small bowel motility. Regrettably, such is not the case for many of our senior patients who celebrate this holiday. If one takes a bolus of matzoh and places it in the intestine of an octogenarian who is mildly dehydrated, one has a theological recipe for a surgical disaster.

That is because, after traveling the eighteen feet to the terminal ileum, matzoh assumes (in the intestine of the dehydrated) the consistency of Spackle™. Rabbis refer to matzoh as the "bread of affliction," a theological reminder of the days of bondage. Working surgeons, however, refer to it as the "bread of obstruction."

"A clear relationship between bowel obstructions and Passover has been commented on at many Matrix Conferences."

Elderly people, already dehydrated, eat large masses of matzoh. It becomes concretized and forms, what pathologists refer to in their reports as an "inspissated, concretized mass of partially digested ritual cracker which has assumed the contour of a sphere impacted in the ileo-cecal valve."* Typically seen on the fourth day of Passover, these patients will appear in the emergency room with a small bowel obstruction. My favorite intern question is: "What is the most common cause of small bowel obstruction in the person with no previous surgery four days into Passover?"

Fortunately, savvy surgeons, rich in the ethnic diversity of their communities can make this diagnosis. This is important since the treatment is always non-surgical. Hydration, avoidance of matzoh and the gradual resumption of clear liquids usually cure this type of obstruction. Any surgical service worth its weight in suture will have at least three or four matzoh bowel obstructions on its service during the Passover holiday.

* See pathology report 84-S #344567 of April 15th 1998 submitted as "obstructing foreign body of ileum."

Matrix Lesson 12

The patient will never
buck at the right time

Matrix discussions will often include facts that do not necessarily show up in an operative report. Some of these facts are problems that occurred during the case. These facts may come to light in the conference setting.

A frequent event is what is referred to as "bucking." Lay people assume that the only bucking going on in this country occurs during rodeos as *meshugennah* people sit astride angry bulls and try to hang on so they can make the 11pm ESPN highlights.

Au contraire! Bucking goes on every day in another other place - in the operating room. Bucking occurs when, during the operation, the patient does, what I refer to as the "D'Arcangelo herky-jerky." So named because Marianne D'Arcangelo, one night, in 1962, danced with me in a manner which sustained my adolescent fantasies up until last year.

"I encourage observation and research among my colleagues to help me find a situation when the patient is bucking at the 'right time.'"

Bucking is an undulating jerk ending with a spasmodic series of contractions. This usually happens during the operation at a time when the patient is supposed to be totally paralyzed and is theoretically unable to move. Lay readers may conjure up horrible scenes of "waking up during the anesthesia." My anesthetic colleagues and I assure you that this is not the case.

Bucking is a primordial reflex appearing in the early part of consciousness, kind of like having dinner with your in-laws. The conscious being of the patient has no recollection, nor does any harm arise from this activity. To the operating surgeon, however, it is annoying and disruptive.

When bucking occurs, surgeons usually look at the anesthetist and, with a soft voice and in a calm manner in keeping with the 1932 Surgery-Anesthesia Peace Agreement of Geneva, say: "The patient is bucking at the wrong time!"

I have thought about this statement for a long time. Why not just say "The patient is bucking"? Adding "the wrong time" is misleading, since it assumes that there is a "right time" to buck.

I encourage observation and research among my colleagues to help me find a situation when the patient is bucking at the "right time." If a patient in your presence ever bucks at the "right" time, please contact me for preparation of a case report.

Matrix Lesson 13

The thrill of avoiding a complication that has befallen the patient of a colleague insures that your patient will experience the same complication within two weeks

I have noticed a certain current in the River of Surgical Fate that assures that any glee one may feel at having avoided a certain trouble, assures that that trouble will come his way. We have all felt that little ripple feeling behind the left ventricle as the resident is presenting an anastomotic leak on the service of a competing colleague.

The Germans have a wonderful word for that feeling - *schadenfreude*. Literally, this means "dark joy." It is the slight flicker of joy that one experiences when an untoward event happens to someone else. It is not purely a bad feeling, nor should the ethicists among my readers take it to heart as a detestable quality of surgeons. It is a natural human feeling. I believe it is the gateway to true compassion.

But let us imagine that this complication has befallen a colleague with whom you hold in low esteem. Let us assume that the complication befell a colleague's patient - the very same patient you saw on a moment's notice who eventually dismissed you as the attending surgeon.

Yes, the very same patient who called you several times and met with you in your office on six occasions with many family members. The same patient who called the county medical society to check your credentials, and, oh yes, the same patient who caused the ruckus in your waiting room because you were a half-hour late for the office. This is that patient.

Your colleague - he's the guy who has berated you at the Matrix Conference for years. He, in fact, is your toughest competitor and a person whose very existence is eroding into your already diminishing patient base.

"Experienced surgeons know that any joy in another's surgical misfortune will deliver the same misfortune to him."

Let us look at the dynamics of the complication with that background.

The complication is presented, or you learn of it. For just one millisecond, putting the case in context, there is a glimmer of having been the target of a horrible situation that was headed for you and has missed the mark, striking someone else. This reaction is perfectly normal: "Whew. I'm glad it wasn't my patient." But that is where it should end.

If it does not end there - if the surgeon relishes the situation, mainly for the torment of his colleague, it is certain that such a complication will head his way within two weeks. This is just a fact of medical life. The gods of surgery giveth and the gods of surgery taketh away.

You will not find a discussion of this in any textbook of surgery. Experienced surgeons know that any joy in another's surgical misfortune will deliver the same misfortune to him.

Matrix Lesson 14

Never begin a comment at the Matrix Conference with "In my experience..." or "That's a research interest of mine!"

The Matrix Conference is theater. The actors are the attending surgeons and the resident-presenters. The script is the history of the complication. The audience is the division of surgery. There is a stage. When participants are recognized by the moderator, they speak as main characters. Sometimes, their introductory remarks give insight into that which will predictably follow.

Certain remarks are shopworn phrases in surgery that are tipoffs to ignorance. Perhaps the most frequent is: "In my experience ..." Much of what the surgeon labels "experience" is a pastiche of misinformation, prejudice, half-truth (one never knows which half) and surgical myth. The fact that some people rely on these comments to bolster arguments or to make points is, to the knowledgeable surgeon, laughable.

"In my experience" is most often used when the scientific, logical and orderly principles of clinical surgery have been shown to play no role in the surgeon's decision-making processes. Backed against a wall of logic, sweating as he confronts his colleagues, when asked to explain himself, he feebly mutters to the assemblage: "In my experience ..." The argument is then lost. The political equivalent of this phrase is "in the interest of national security."

Surgeons use a variety of other ploys to generate an aura of intellectual sophistication. Of all the ploys used, my personal favorite is: "That's a research interest of mine." I understand the role of research in surgery (Summertime employment for the children of influential surgeons) and I recognize the valuable debt we owe to surgical research (the Teflon-coated electrocautery tip). Yet the number of people who invoke a personal research interest far outnumbers the amount of research going on. Do these people have laboratories in their garages? Do these people fly to the NIH for seminars and just tell people they are going skiing in Aspen. It is as if every attending surgeon, during a discussion, becomes Louis Pasteur!

"Certain remarks are shopworn phrases in surgery that are tipoffs to ignorance. Perhaps the most frequent is, 'In my experience....'"

If you are doing legitimate research, please discuss it and hopefully benefit some patient, but don't throw "research interests" around the Matrix Conference as if those interests are your *raison d'être*.

Save these terms for the following situations:

- A third year medical student lecture.
- A group of new internists.
- A cocktail party for lay people.
- Your in-laws.

In my experience, these terms are most effective in these situations.

Matrix Lesson 15

Never criticize your chief resident
or your partner in a group setting

I have recently noticed an increasingly contentious relationship evolving among surgical residents. This same phenomenon is mirrored on a higher level among attending surgical partners.

I came through my surgical training in the days of strict deference to authority. My chief resident was a demi-god. The attending surgeon was a god.

If the chief resident sent me to do something - I did it. It was his triumphal year and he was due the respect and dedication I gave him. When I went into practice, my senior partners (employers) were also gods. They had paid their surgical dues. I had not. It was that simple. I never questioned them, challenged them or touched them.

I have noticed a gradual erosion of the status of the chief resident. Perhaps it is due to today's culture. Maybe it is the result of a better medical education in which students got in touch with their inner self. I do not know. This change is nowhere more clearly seen than when a chief resident is criticized, questioned or challenged by one of the residents on his service.

For example: the chief resident is presenting a case at the Matrix Conference. The discussion is ending. A junior resident raises his hand, is recognized and says: "Dr. Phelps, wasn't there a real question about the viability of the left colon?" Or, even worse: "I think the hematocrit was 23%, not 37% as you said." Today, these questions are answered respectfully and logically by the chief resident. The questions, though legitimate and thought-provoking, can be embarrassing to the chief.

If I had asked such a question in a group setting, I would have been sent to medical records and barred from the operating room for a week. I never asked such questions out of respect to the chief resident and the knowledge that one day I would be standing there challenged by the attending staff. The last thing I would want, or would expect, would be an assault from one of my own.

"Surgery is a team discipline. ..... Analyze, question, opine - but save the criticisms for the corridor, the lounge or the office."

Similarly, I have seen junior partners challenge their senior partners, often in conference settings. I find this unfathomable. A surgical office should, to some degree, be a unified surgical team. At a more practical level, the good name and reputation of the office are singular qualities which are difficult to preserve. Such questioning from within hardly solidifies the reputation of a unified front of surgical excellence.

This issue bridges the gap between surgical loyalty and surgical honesty. This allegiance to chief or partner may sometimes blur the line between the two. It can be a delicate path to tread.

I am not advocating abandoning the lively debate over surgical issues. Nor am I advocating looking the other way. I am advocating the judicious timing of questions, especially in a group setting.

Surgery is a team discipline. The *esprit de corp* of that team is a fragile element which can be destroyed with a single volley. Analyze, question, opine - but save the criticisms for the corridor, the lounge or the office.

[Note to chief residents - you are the chief - if you say the hematocrit was 35%, then it was 35%!].

[Note to partners - the next time you have the urge to ask that probing question, remember that this is the same guy who drove in at 03:00 Hrs. to bail you out. Resist the temptation. Let it pass!].

Matrix Lesson 16

The likelihood that a surgical case will remain in your office is inversely proportional to the amount of office energy expended in arranging that case

Or $L = 1/T$, where L = likelihood that the case is yours; T = office time spent on arranging the case, i.e. physician discussion and exam of patient, calls to referring physician, discussion with patient's family, secretarial time in arranging scheduling, preparation and surgical arrangements.

The Matrix Conference is an open assembly of all surgeons in the division. In today's world, because of insurance plans or patient preference, it is increasingly common for one surgeon to evaluate a patient, yet have another surgeon perform the surgery.

Although it may shock some of my internal medical colleagues, the evaluation and assessment, the scheduling and arranging, the co-ordination, the cognitive activity, planning and preparation that goes into a surgical case is considerable.

Most internists have this vision of the surgeon, waiting in his office to fill the eternally available operating theater. The concept of a busy surgeon evaluating and arranging is strangely foreign to them.

"Spend the time, but never assume that this time will result in the case staying with you."

Surgeons vary in their ability to spend time with patients and to generate that timeless devotion to the patient seen only on various prime time medical shows. The exigencies of the day often are not conducive to the gentle and leisurely evaluation we all hope we could perform.

Ms. Nancy Senter, my office manager for twenty-two years, re-enforced the formulation of Matrix Lesson #16 when, after scheduling a complicated pelvic tumor case for the third time after the second office visit for family discussions, looked me squarely in the eye and said: "You will never do this case."

With stunning predictability, three days later a curt message was left on my answering service: "Cancel my surgery, I've gone elsewhere."

Curiously, there are days when the patient gets evaluated, but not with the time commitment they expect or you would like to deliver. A sleep-deprived surgeon two hours late for the office with an early evening case pending cannot be the model of the meticulous and diplomatic consultant. The job gets done with expertise and concern, but in a somewhat hurried manner. No matter what the problem, if this scenario involves the scheduling of a case, it is likely that that patient will stay with you and adore you. For some inexplicable reason, this consult results in an adoring patient who would follow you through a war.

Never assume that there is payback for time spent. For some reason this is particularly true of breast disease. Lengthy discussions of intraductal carcinoma, lobular carcinoma *in situ* and other controversial areas result in the proper surgical procedure scheduled and performed expertly .... by someone else!

This is Lesson #16. Spend the time, but never assume that this time will result in the case staying with you.

Matrix Lesson 17

The least essential operating room
supplies are always over-stocked

"Obverse of Law #17: the most
essential operating room
supplies are always back-
ordered."

The issue of operating room systems and supplies will
come up at a Matrix Conference. Occasionally a
surgeon will frankly state that what he needed was just
not available. There is a valuable lesson here.

Somewhere in the *Big Book of Operating Room
Administration* is the chapter titled "The Verschimmelt
Philosophy of Ordering Operating Room Supplies." This
philosophy states that infrequently requested expensive

supplies must be over-stocked while oft-needed inexpensive supplies must be back-ordered.

If you need chromate impregnated 8-0 schmearolon on an Italian needle, you can get it immediately because it is over-stocked. Somebody, back in 1987, ordered nine boxcarloads of it. It is available row after row on the supply cart near the surgeons' lounge. Some surgeon had an affair with the schmearolon sales lady which resulted in a dramatic over-supply of this useless suture.

However, if you need a new blade for the Balfour retractor, a new electrocautery tip, or lowly 3-0 chromic suture, it is out of stock. It is out of stock because of the philosophic underpinning of operating room administration mentioned above. It is out of stock because it is an essential item.

Why is this and how did this administrative principle evolve? To understand this we must trace the history of operating room administration and focus on the Germanic phase of the late eighteen hundreds. We must discuss the activities of Theodor Billroth the great surgical innovator. His operating rooms were laboratories of surgical innovation in which he demanded that new products be developed and that new procedures be invented. It was Billroth's theory that if everything was available, there would be no stimulus to surgical innovation or invention. *Therefore, it was his edict that surgeons be denied what they needed on a daily basis as a means of stimulating their surgical creativity.*

Why should a surgeon get what he wants every day? What better way to stimulate his creative surgical mind than to deny him what he needs! This worked very well in Billroth's Vienna. It led to many innovations. Unfortunately, however, for the working surgeon of today, this principle is outdated. Nevertheless, it remains a central theme in schools of operating room administration.

One other historical explanation for Billroth's practices might be his investment in several Bavarian research and development firms in the late 1870s. In a frighteningly obvious conflict of interest, he ordered seldom used supplies exclusively from the Sondrgeblick Gesellschaft, a firm in which he was a limited partner. This event is one of the darker chapters in the history of surgical academia. Its effects linger today as prominent surgeons invest in instrument companies and then badger helpless nurse-managers into ordering seldom needed supplies.

Billroth cemented this operating room principle forever when he married his own operating room administrator, Frau Gribeness. As you may know he had seven sons. When asked why such a surgical innovator had such a large family, Billroth is said to have replied: "I needed condoms, but they were on back-order!"

Matrix Lesson 18

Always listen to your haustra

The hallmark of the medical conference is the interruption - the beeper, the cell-phone, the overhead page, the coming and going as physicians attend to the ill. Sometimes those interruptions arise from physiology rather than from professional obligations. I refer, of course, to the primal urges (or at least two of the primal urges). Although a discussion of a surgical complication is important, I encourage all participants - presenter or audience, resident or attending - to respond to that urge.

Shortly after the primitive hindgut migrated from the primitive midgut and said good-bye to the primitive foregut, the haustra appeared. Teleologically, phenomenologically and certainly histologically, these evanescent saccules evolved to fill a basic need - the ability to control excretion as well as to employ fluoroscopy technicians.

While the main job of colonic control is the ultra-sophisticated gas/solid differentiator of the primitive ano-rectum, that control is complimented by the haustra. These saccular outpouchings of the colon got their name in an interesting manner. The *haustrum* was a primitive machine for drawing water. It was a series of cups placed on a moving belt which would draw water up from a stream. The ancient anatomists viewed the sacculations of the colon which when spread out looked like this machine. The sacculations were then referred to as haustra.

"The underlying source of **unhappiness** among the surgical **staff** of most general surgical services is a **denial** of the **haustral** effect."

One of my seminal experiences in surgery was the first time I laid eyes on Horace Davenport's masterpiece *The Physiology of the Digestive Tract*. There, on page two hundred and fifty-three was the sentence that sent me on my general surgical career: "... the lips of the anus vibrate like the double reed of a bassoon, sounding a low-pitched note." (Yearbook Medical Publishers, Fourth Edition, Chicago, 1977).

How could any physician resist the siren call of the discipline of gastrointestinal surgery after reading those words? The haustra contribute timbre to that note. The haustra evolved over millenia. Who dares deny their will?

And yet we do. We who so devotedly study the haustra and operate upon them, deny their daily call. The underlying source of unhappiness among the surgical staff of most general surgical services is a denial of the haustral effect. This is why the chief of surgery is always frowning. This denial is a contributing factor to the development of colon cancer, as well as various international conflicts. The reluctance of busy surgeons to respond immediately to haustral distension is an endemic problem, one which the American Society of Surgeons is only now addressing. The surgical day does not allow the proper response to the haustra. The ursurgeon responded by immediately crouching behind a rock.

But then civilization came along and so did surgical schedules and rounds with the chief. Where does it say in the Hippocratic Oath that each oath-taker must disregard this most basic of biologic urges and go one-on-one with his or her haustra?

I instruct every participant in the Matrix Conference that the inexplicable disappearance of a fellow resident is, in fact, an in-depth testament to that resident's knowledge of colon physiology.

Always listen to your haustra - even in mid-sentence when talking to a family, while pointing out to the intern the folly of removing the T-tube on postoperative day #2 or when presenting a case at the Matrix Conference.

Knowledgeable surgeons will understand your hasty exit.

Matrix Lesson 19

The operation is over when the patient is eating a cheeseburger and can't remember your name

I am always amazed at the youthful naiveté demonstrated by some surgeons and almost all residents by post-procedure celebrations. "Great case! Fantastic case!" These post-surgical comments tempt fate and demonstrate a complete disregard for the postoperative period. This is a sign of the inexperienced. I call it premature euphoriation - high-fiving and jubilation happening before it is justified. Such activity almost assures a lethal complication. Premature euphoriation reflects a lack of understanding, not so much of the physiology of surgery as of the spirit of surgery.

Eighty percent of cases which have such post-surgical celebrations will experience a complication. These celebrations are particularly dangerous in general surgery - the most demanding and clinically challenging field of surgery. Anastomotic healing problems, bleeding, postoperative bowel obstructions, intra-abdominal abscess formation - each of these is hiding behind every flippant comment regarding the "smoothness" of the operation.

If I were a mythologist (and listening to some of the resident case presentations I am rapidly becoming one), I would create the mythologic god of postoperative courses. He would be called Hubris the Great. He would be a man with a leaking anastomosis in his right hand and a CT scan showing a sub-phrenic abscess in his left hand. Slung over his shoulder would be arrows dipped in humility and respect.

Each arrow would have a small picture of the heart of the surgeon who performed the operation. A picture of Hubris the Great would hang in every surgeon's lounge. Hubris the Great would be on guard for postoperative celebrations. His presence would deter them.

"Premature euphoriation reflects a lack of understanding, not so much of the physiology of surgery as of the spirit of surgery."

Operations are part of a continuum which, though it may wind down, never really ends. The operation is over when the patient is healed, back to as functional a level as possible and when the memory of his surgery (and his surgeon) is fading. The operation is over when the chances of a postoperative complication become remote. The operation is over when that wonderful sense of well-being envelopes the patient, i.e. when the patient is at home watching Sportscenter. The operation is over when your office calls for a missed appointment because the patient is feeling too well to come back. The operation is over when the patient orders the double-chili cheeseburger with a side of curly-fries and his wife says: "Hey what was the name of that surgeon?" and he honestly cannot remember.

Then the operation is over. Then the celebration can begin.

Matrix Lesson 20

The slashed skin incision handled by delayed primary closure in a trauma case with a perforated colon will heal perfectly

"Obverse of Law #20: the planned skin incision for an elective case on a colleague's wife laboriously closed with 9-0 nylon will heal as if by secondary intent."

The advent of digital photography has enhanced Matrix Conference presentations. Wedded with presentation graphics, the audience can view the incision and the operative field. At subsequent conferences the audience can witness the follow-up of the case.

There is extreme variation in the final appearance of healed skin incisions. Some perverse law of nature dictates that the greater the care and the more ideal circumstances which exist in general surgery, the greater the likelihood of a horrific scar.

I have planned incisions and have repaired them in multiple layers with the greatest devotion to plastic surgical technique. I have followed Langer's lines. I have avoided the dreaded bevel or the even more dreaded skive. I have applied the proper pressure at precisely a ninety-degree angle to the skin. In short, I have poured years of expertise and allegiance to the scar gods into the elective incision. Sadly, for me and for the patient, the result often is that which might be mistaken for a knife fight in South Boston.

It is important, in the elective setting, that patients understand that an acceptable scar, although enhanced by some basic surgical concepts, is very much an individual trait.

I have also thrown prep solution on dying patients and slashed my way into the abdomen in an effort to save a life. These incisions have been left open. For some unknown surgical reason, these patients have been frequently rewarded with a thin, barely perceptible pencil line for a scar.

These scar scenarios are the body's way of reminding the surgeon that other factors are always at work in surgery. It provides a leveling effect for surgeons who are overwhelmed by their own expertise.

Juxtaposed, the two situations outlined above led to Matrix Lesson #20.

Matrix Lesson 21

If a patient develops a postoperative problem, consider the anatomic complications of the operation before any other *vercackte** diagnoses

---

One time I got a midnight call from a urologist. He called about a patient with lower abdominal pain three days after a trans-urethral prostatectomy. The urologist told me that the patient had appendicitis.

I told him that I was the King of Sweden.

Here we have a grown man - a urologist of wide repute. He takes a silver shaft with a laser light at the end of it. He activates 4500 Joule/watts/second on the lining of the prostate and examines the bladder. He then removes the instrument of his will.

How is it that his thought process led him to appendicitis, exclusive of the more probable anatomic complications of his own procedure?

* Vercackte - Yiddish adjective which, politely translated, means illogical or nonsensical.

Call me a wild and wacky consultant, but it is perfectly logical to assume that the problem arose from the initial surgery. I raised the issue of a perforated bladder with extravasation, but was told simply that "we don't see that after prostatectomy." I replied, that William of Occam** would never have agreed with him. William of Occam stated that things ought not be made unnecessarily complicated. Or, once the most logical explanation of an event has been formulated, there is little need to invoke other explanations.

At that hour, the urologist was not impressed with William of Occam. He hung up the phone and called another consultant. A cystogram had been ordered which showed [*mirabile victu*], a perforation of the bladder.

> "... it is perfectly logical to assume that the problem arose from the initial surgery."

The case was eventually presented at the Matrix Conference. After a circuitous resident presentation on the differential diagnosis of supra-pubic pain, I had the very enjoyable experience of explaining to my department the influence of William of Occam on the human bladder.

Why surgeons conjure up non-anatomic explanations for plausible anatomic problems is a topic for another paper. Left lower quadrant pain after a sigmoid colectomy (anastomotic leak); rectal pain and fullness after a ruptured appendix (pelvic abscess); right upper quadrant pain after a laparoscopic cholecystectomy (bile leak) - think anatomically! Once the likelihood of an anatomically-related problem lessens, then you can start thinking like an internist.

I am tempted to dredge up the old saw: "If you hear hoofbeats, think of horses," but I sound more elegant discussing William of Occam.

** See Matrix Lesson #36.

Matrix Lesson 22

Academic surgical discussions are allowed from 08:00 Hrs. to 18:00 Hrs.

I have always been annoyed by those who assume that just because they are awake, so too is the rest of the world.

Spare me the long-winded meandering case presentation at 03:45 Hrs. Do not regale me with the patient's cousin's history of porphyria. Do not mention the recent trip to Venezuela with the consumption of tainted cassaba.

Be precise. Be brief. Be to the point - especially in the middle of the night. When it became obvious to me that surgical sleep deprivation was a national health threat I wrote a landmark article called "A Plea for the Medical Precis."* This essay was a request to the medical world to boil down the essentials of a case, particularly after hours.

* Gordon LA. A Plea for the Medical Précis. JAMA 1982; 258(11): 1300.

I was instantly reviled as a medical nihilist. I had fulfilled the stereotype of the surgeon interested only in the procedure. In this case the stereotype was true for the after hours consult. This led to the formulation of Matrix Lesson #22 - legitimate hours for academic discourse.

This lesson is quite simple. Get into the habit, during off hours, of developing a précis of the case. The précis was a difficult drill in high school English class. We were limited to five sentences to summarize a novel or a short story. Working on the précis develops two valuable skills for the physician: an appreciation for the short story and the ability to separate the medical wheat from the medical chaff.

"Be precise. Be brief. Be to the point - especially in the middle of the night."

Internists can take the chaff and have a seminar. Surgeons will take the wheat and will bake a loaf of medical care.

The working surgeon has basically one question in the middle of the night: is he needed for a surgical judgment or is he needed to perform surgery?

I will let the professors discourse at those hours on the differential diagnoses, the subtle historical points and the fascinating permutations of retractile mesenteritis. I will let the professors educate medical residents on the simplest points of surgical care. I will let the professors year after year outline the most basic aspects of a work-up of right lower quadrant pain.

I prefer sleep. I am a union academician - eight to six, no weekends. If you call me at that hour, have the case thought out and well-prepared. If you do not, please call someone else.

Matrix Lesson 23

If the scrub nurses mumble during the sponge count, get a film

Much has been written about the retained sponge. It is a fertile area for litigation. These cases are presented at the Matrix Conference since every return to the operating room is discussed.

Here is the usual scenario. The case has gone well. You are closing the abdomen. The final sponge count has begun. Then it begins. Quietly, out of the corner of your consciousness, the scrub nurse and the circulating nurse intrude.

They begin to mumble. Much like the Dick Tracy character of the same name, their conversation sounds like this: "... mmmm, lap pad ..... four CT needles .... under the table .... seven, eight, nine .... I thought ten ... mmm ... Did Sally? Floor ... where? ... mmm ... was that Michelle or Donna ... mble, mble, mmm."

After a surgeon hears this mumbling, the following exchange occurs:

Surgeon: "Is our count o.k.?"
Nurse: [No reply].
Surgeon: "Ladies, is our count o.k.?"
Nurse: Pause. "Yes. Just a minute."

At this point, the fascial closure is almost complete. Some surgeons, pause, re-open and check for laparotomy pads, sponges or clamps. Most surgeons continue their closure.

Five minutes pass.

Surgeon: "How are we doing? Is the count correct?"
Nurse: "Mmmm ... 3, 4, 5, ... 9, 10 ... Was that a pop-off? ... Millie relieved me, went to second lunch and said three laparotomy pads not four ... Mmmm ... 2, 3, 4, ... Alice went to first break."

At this point in the never ending assault on surgeons' coronaries, there is only one logical move - obtain an abdominal film before the patient leaves the operating theater.

I have a great deal of respect for the scrub nurses and circulating nurses of the world. They are expert, dedicated and precise in their craft. Yet, the system of lunch, coffee and break relief often interferes with the sponge-counting aspects of an operation. Somewhere between second lunch, third coffee and fourth break (as mandated by the nurses' Union) can arise inconsistencies in the sponge count.

"Any mumbling, concern, irregularity, or less than forceful assessment of the sponge or needle count should lead to an abdominal X-ray."

Those inconsistencies can be quite unsettling to the operating surgeon, not to mention the serosa of the left colon as it embarks on foreplay with a laparotomy pad.

Any mumbling, concern, irregularity, or less than forceful assessment of the sponge or needle count should lead to an abdominal X-ray. After viewing the film, the mumbling may proceed all the way to third lunch, or fourth coffee, or maybe even into second break.

Matrix Lesson 24

The intern you grill the hardest about a specific topic will have a Ph.D. in that topic

---

The Matrix Conference is an active give-and-take between resident and attending. The attending assumes he knows more than the resident, particularly about the topic at hand.

Beware! This is not always the case, as Lesson #24 will demonstrate.

I enjoy questioning interns in the operating room. I am short, not very intelligent and often sleep-deprived. Mix these three elements together, add an unending supply of interns, and one can see what joy it gives me to make a former USC linebacker quake in my presence.

Matrix Lesson #24 addresses the issue of the time-honored practice of asking questions during surgery or on rounds.

"However, the more one presses an intern on a subject ... the greater the likelihood that the intern or resident will have a doctorate in that area."

I am a devotee of the Socratic method of surgical education. Surgery is very much a "what-if" specialty. Surgery demands instant recall of fact and thoughtful planning of action. Surgery often involves making rapid decisions under tight circumstances. I try to emulate the onslaught of surgical pathology with my ever escalating questioning of interns and residents.

However, the more one presses an intern on a subject; the more one tries to expose an intern's ignorance about a specific topic; the more glee an attending derives from pursuing a line of questions - *the greater the likelihood that the intern or resident will have a doctorate in that area.*

Interns are different nowadays. Many of them are not the techno-geek-fast-track-grinder that my generation was before applying to medical school. Some of them actually have lived a bit before entering training. They come to surgery with broad life and educational experiences. These experiences have educated them in many areas well beyond my own experiences.

Some personal examples:

- I am grilling the intern on the embryology of the extra-hepatic biliary tree.
  She has a Ph.D. in anatomy and embryology from Northwestern University.
- I am grilling the resident on the physics of the obstructed colon.
  He has a Ph.D. in Physics from Berkeley.

- I am grilling the intern on the events surrounding Carl Yastrezmski's last at-bat.
  He played Triple A ball for the Red Sox in Pawtucket.
- I am grilling the intern on the name and condition of the patient who was Billroth's first gastrectomy.
  His father is a surgeon in Vienna.

Nothing brings my colleagues greater joy than when, mid-sentence during an intra-operative discussion, the resident meekly replies: "Doctor Gordon, I did my doctoral thesis on that at Yale."

I retreat to the surgeons' lounge, lick my attending wounds, then rejoin the operating team.

I have never really mastered Matrix Lesson #24.

Matrix Lesson 25

Never unfasten the brassiere of an elderly immigrant woman during evaluation of a breast problem

I have witnessed very few complications of breast surgery at the Matrix Conference. Nevertheless, there is one potential complication that may occur. It is a unique surgical complication that may hurt the surgeon, not the patient.

The formulation of Matrix Law #25 is not racial or ethnic profiling. As a youth, I remember my mother helping my grandmother into a contraption to get her ready for high profile social functions in Haverhill, Massachusetts, in the mid-fifties (the weekly Mah-Jhong game).

Those juvenile Freudian memories center about my diminuitive mother attempting to encase my corpulent grandmother into a contraption supported with laces and whale bones. This is the basis for Matrix Lesson #25.

The Russians kept up with the United States for a long time in every field of national life, except brassiere development. Recently, major metropolitan areas throughout the country have seen increasing numbers of Russian immigrants. Many of these immigrants are elderly women who are in need of breast exams and follow-up of breast problems.

Something horrible must have happened to the Russian lingerie business in the 1930s through to the 1950s. It is as if the Kommissar of Structural Bridge and Road Development set out plans and those plans wound up on the desk of the Kommissar of Underwear Development.

"Do not attempt to defuse the bra unsupervised! The surgeon should ask a family member to help."

Because of this historical mix-up, the underwear of older Russian women has hooks, laces, snapping mechanisms, configuring compression bands, cantilevers, struts, Y-braces, laces, straps, strings, thongs, cross supports, fornices, finials, tenons, mortises and various metallic objects designed to compress the upper thorax. It is amazing that any Russian grandmother can breathe!

Often, because of language problems, the woman will not understand that she must disrobe to allow a full exam. This means that the unsuspecting surgeon may enter an examining room and be confronted with such a women wearing a Russian bra.

Do not attempt to defuse the bra unsupervised!

The surgeon should ask a family member to help. Only an intimate knowledge of the device assures its safe removal. These devices can be treacherous. No surgeon should unfurl one unless he is familiar with its intricacies.* Once the support garment has been removed, the surgeon can then *safely* proceed with his standard breast examination.

Tell your scheduling nurse to allow at least one-half hour for re-application of the garment as family members grunt, groan and re-apply the device. They may need heavy equipment to do this. Arrangements should be made with the office building's service staff to plan for this eventuality. This is usually a three man (or woman) task.

There is some evidence to support the theory that the actual cause of the Tsungutska forest blast in 1908 was the surreptitious disrobing of the Czar's paramour who was wearing such a mammary support device.

* See Somlensk V, Vitrahoutovich R. Forced Blast Entropy from Accidental Release of Soviet Mammary Supports in the Office Setting. *Acta Mammographa Sovietska* 1968; 6(4): 123-45.

Matrix Lesson 26

Never use the grammatically correct plural
of pancreatitis, diverticulitis or mesenteritis

The giggle center of the human brain is indestructible.
Posterior to the limbus, just lateral to the rhinencephalon,
and underneath the area controlling social
consciousness - the giggle center allows humans (even
tenured professors of surgery), at any age and under any
circumstance, to giggle under certain circumstances.

Psychologic development, education, training and
social mores cannot interfere with its function - the
generation of a giggle at an amusing event. The giggle
center serves a useful social and evolutionary purpose.
Although ablated at birth in most department chairmen,
it continues to have a great influence on surgery and on
medical education.

Regrettably, there are few giggle-generating events in
medicine today. The full-frontal assault on our profession

from many detractors has made us a bit defensive and a bit humorless. We must seek out humor and elements of our professional life at which to laugh.

When we are young, we giggle in school and in church. When we are old, we giggle for no apparent reason, usually alone in the doctors' parking lot or at funerals.

Giggling is healthy. Giggling is man's way of recognizing ultimate contradictions even at the most serious of times.

The major giggle-generating event for literate physicians, is a colleague's attempt to use the grammatically correct plural forms of the suffix -itis. One may logically ask, "How can a plural noun be funny?" This is my genius. I will tell you.

Since the suffix -itis is Greek in origin, the proper plural, becomes -itides. Because the central accent creates a slang term ingrained in our culture, no-one can say or listen to this plural without thinking of this particular term.

I said no-one!

Whether you are the Fothergill Professor of Surgery in London, the Chairman of Feminist Medical Studies or a rotating student from Chicago, no-one can think of anything but the slang meaning of this accented syllable.

"Giggling is healthy."

I suspect that most people who use the proper plural form are testing the audience rather than demonstrating their classical education. I am not ashamed to admit that I violate Lesson #26 quite frequently.

I usually use these proper plurals as a test of the restraint and demeanor of residents or colleagues who do not know me. Ex-clergy, Ivy

League graduates and exchange students wrestling with English are particularly ripe targets for me, usually on rounds and most assuredly in a group setting.

Giggling at the proper use of these plurals is a human constant. Anyone who can control themselves during the use of these proper plurals, or during the repetition of these words is a strong individual - most assuredly life-less and devoid of humor - but strong nevertheless.

They are the same people who do not think of the Lone Ranger when they hear the William Tell overture.

Matrix Lesson 27

Have, at the very least, a passing acquaintance with surgical history

The difference between a profession and a trade is that a profession has a greater sense of history woven into its daily activities.

When I was younger, I always told the residents that the first sign of senility in a surgeon is when he demonstrates an interest in surgical history. I was wrong, because I was a closet historian and was ashamed to admit it. I enjoyed reading about those who were in the business long before I was.

Medicine has the most interesting history of any profession. Excluding various ranches in Nevada, medicine is, in fact, the oldest profession.

There was medicine before there was anything. When a Neanderthal got a headache, he looked for medicine.

The Spanish Armada needed medicine. And always, men and women were there to provide it. Among the blood-letters, clysterers and herb doctors, some very interesting people stood out. Since we are in the same profession, we owe a great debt to them. It is only proper that we be acquainted with them.

We stand on the shoulders of medical giants. If those giants on whom we stand were to look up they would recognize two things: we have gained a lot of weight and, there is gender equality in medicine today. For these reasons, we have an obligation to study surgical history.

"Reading surgical history makes one an educated surgeon, as well as a trained surgeon."

I expect a basic knowledge of surgical history from any resident involved in the weekly Matrix Conference. I expect a more refined knowledge from my colleagues. This explains why I always sit alone in the doctor's eating area.

Reading surgical history is fun. Reading surgical history is interesting. Reading surgical history makes one an educated surgeon, as well as a trained surgeon.

To be culturally literate in surgical history, one should be acquainted with the following names:

Hippocrates	Halsted	Galen
Halston	Twiggy	McDowell (Ephraim and Roddy)
Sushruta	McPherson (Elle and Lester)	Theophrastus Bombastus
Beaumont	Ambrose Paré	Guy LaFleur

Bassini	Marcus Welby	Rossini
Marcus Allen	Fellini	Marcus Aurelius
Scallopini	Priapus	Billroth
Bill Roth	Bill Buckner	Virchow
Howser	Horchow	Prof. Irwin Corey
Charles Bingham	Sam Sump	Penrose
Fitz	Forrest Gump	Hieronymous Gram
Blalock	Mr. H&E	Jackson and Pratt
Frau Blücher	Bialystock and Blum	Taussig
Montana and Rice	Kanavel	Starzl
Knievel	Sabiston	Knadle
Yastrezemski	Wöffler	Gordon
Paracelsus	Heller	Buttafuoco

"... we have an obligation to study surgical history."

We are part of a grand tradition. It began with the first person to apply pressure to the bleeding wound of a loved one. It continues through our work today. This rich history makes our work more interesting. A basic knowledge of this history is a testament to the respect we have for our profession and our forbears.

Matrix Lesson 28

The patient will always be given
a drug to which he is allergic

"Corollary of Law #28: the administration of that drug will have no effect."

Medication errors are a major focus of current efforts at patient safety. Great strides are being made in this area with the advent of bar-coding (medications and patients) and computer-generated drug warnings. But no system is perfectly foolproof.

It is impossible to be admitted to a hospital, to be checked in by the nurses, to be evaluated by the intern and to be screened by the attending surgeon without being looked squarely in the eye and being asked: "Are you allergic to any medications?"

Stickers are affixed to the chart, notations are made in capital letters on typed consults, nurses' notes are emblazoned with various neon and psychedelically-colored stickers that a drug allergy is present. The question is again asked prior to checking into the operating theater, proceeding to specialized tests or during interviews by other consultants.

Yet somehow, magically and with predictable regularity, that specific drug is administered to the patient during the hospitalization.

How this occurs is very interesting. The analysis of this occurrence has occupied a good deal of my time. It is, as we say in the internist's lounge, "a research interest of mine." (See Matrix Lesson #14).

The drug may be given by a cross-covering resident who does not know the patient and who is called upon to make a judgment in an emergent situation. The drug may be given by the attending surgeon's partner who must also act in an emergent situation. The patient may fall into a protocol carried out in the operating theater, such as the routine administration of some antibiotics before surgery. Or perhaps the ever cost-conscious pharmacy director may substitute one drug for another.

Despite the safeguards and warnings, and despite the multiple questions and stickers, somehow the drug to which the patient is allergic is administered.

The truly magical aspect of Lesson #28 is its corollary. That aspect is the response of the patient to the drug. That response is ... well ... no response. The drug is administered. It has its desired effect. The patient is none the worse for its administration. No allergy exists.

The reason for these magical twists and turns of medical fate is that what most people consider to be allergies are really not drug allergies. "I am allergic to iodine" usually means intermittent flushing during an IVP. "I am allergic to penicillin" usually means some gastric upset following ingestion. "I am allergic to all the -caines" * usually means some tachycardia or mild flushing after an injection of local anesthetic in a dentist's office.

Matrix Lesson #28 is not a call to disregard the patient's history and real drug allergies.

Lesson #28 is merely an observation which stands as a testament to the resilience of the human organism as it faces a three-pronged attack by disease, those treating the disease and the vagaries of life as a patient in a medical center.

---

* I once examined a priest who said "I am allergic to all the -caines." I then asked "What about the Abels?" He relieved me of my surgical duties and sought additional consultation in the university setting.

Matrix Lesson 29

Never mumble in the operating theater

The English language has evolved over thousands of years. It is a marvelous accomplishment that what were once primordial mud-slugs can now converse and present themselves on afternoon talk shows.

Some of these mud-slugs evolved even further into surgical residents and surgeons. Years of education, rigorous discipline in the art and science of medicine, and years of practice have honed these surgical cortices into intelligent forces.

Why is it then, that some of these brilliant types mumble during surgery? Why is it that these supremely capable physicians, when viewing an operative field filled with the very essence of their craft will say something like: "mmph, sgrst, colon-mmphph, ... phrmp!" or even worse "slmmr, ... office, ... phrmph, ... damn ....."

I was educated by some of the worst mumblers in the business. Here I was, an impressionable resident, trying to learn, trying to pick the surgical pearls off of the operating room floor and what was thrown my way?

Grown men and women mumbling beneath a mask. Fractured words, indistinct syllabic ramblings - the mumbled musings of once brilliant minds.

"Be bold or be ridiculous in your statements, but never mumble!"

It was during my training that I pledged never to mumble. Furthermore, I pledged to dismiss mumblers from my operating theater.

If a resident is asked a question in the operating theater or on rounds ... If a circulating nurse is asked the location of an instrument or piece of equipment ... If the anesthesiologist is asked if there is a problem ... If your colleagues are asked to voice an opinion ... *Be right. Be wrong. Be bold or be ridiculous in your statements, but never mumble!*

Any resident mumbling in my operating theater or at the Matrix Conference is dismissed.

The clearest illustration of the effects of mumbling on the mind of the attending surgeon can be found in the 1984 movie *Amadeus*. This film chronicles the madness of court composer, Salieri, as he is confronted with the genius of Mozart. This movie should be shown to all surgical interns on July 1 of every year.

The opening scene and the closing scene of the movie transport the viewer down the corridor of an insane asylum of the late 1700s. The long corridor tracking shots are littered with the insane, many of whom approach the camera.

Most of these unfortunate beings are mumbling.

Court composer, Salieri, was driven mad by Mozart's genius. It is unlikely that I or any other surgical attending will be driven mad by the genius of a surgical resident. They have too many other maddening qualities, the most prominent of which is intra-operative mumbling.

Any surgeon viewing those two scenes from *Amadeus* will agree that the people lining that corridor were once attending surgeons forced to work with residents or colleagues who mumbled.

Amadeus won seven academy awards. I give it an even higher honor. I use it as an illustration of Matrix Lesson #29: best portrayal of the effects of mumbling on attending surgeons.

Matrix Lesson 30

Misery will follow the surgical *k'enohorah*

After several years in surgery, a surgeon gets to be pretty skillful at analyzing facial expressions. As the Moderator of our Matrix Conference, I have observed the faces of attending surgeons as their complications are being analyzed. Sometimes I note a look of incredulity. This arises from a simple thought: "How could a case that had gone so well turn out so poorly? What happened." Many times there will be no specific surgical-technical answer, which brings us to the *k'enohorah*.

A k'enohorah is an ancient invocation used to ward off ill winds. In surgery, however, this invocation always works in reverse. One gives the surgical k'enohorah by prematurely boasting of success or by reveling in exceptional skill.

Leo Rosten in *The Joys of Yinglish** describes it as an exclamation used to assuage the gods and to avoid tempting them to anger.

In surgery, however, k'enohorah causes the cosmic forces of bad luck to appear. My wife always gives me the reverse k'enohorah when I'm playing blackjack in Las Vegas. I will split 4s, stand on twelves and double on Ace-8s and win every hand. I will win, until she says: "Boy you can do no wrong tonight!"

By definition, she has just given me the k'enohorah. Had she not spoken these words, I will continue to win. Having spoken the words, the k'enorhah has been delivered, and I will lose the next fifteen hands!

This reverse curse can be delivered during surgery also. It is this circumstance that Matrix Lesson #30 addresses. The surgical k'enohorah states simply and clearly that any expression of ease or simplicity surrounding a surgical case will lead to either: a) an unexpected and inextricably difficult intra-operative situation; or b) a horrible postoperative complication.

"In surgery, however, k'enohorah causes the cosmic forces of bad luck to appear."

Situation A arises two hours into a Whipple procedure. The stomach, common duct, pancreas and the Ligament of Treitz are divided. The entire specimen is to the patient's right as you are about to begin the dissection of the gland off of the portal vein. The smell of an impending coffee break wafts through the operating room.

At this point in time, a cheery voice, usually that of the anesthesiologist, blares from the top of the drapes: "Gee, we'll be out of here in an hour!"

* The best descriptions of the k'enohorah are in *The Joys of Yinglish* by Leo Rosten. New York: Penguin Books, 1989: 289.

This glib comment assures a horrible turn of events. Albeit unintentionally, the k'enohorah has been delivered. A laceration of the portal vein, tumor fixation to the uncinate, unexplained intra-operative hypotension - you name it and it will happen. All because of this naive expression of good fortune.

Situation B addresses the curse in the postoperative state. At the conclusion of a low anterior resection, someone will state: "That was great. He'll sail." This assures an anastomotic leak, a pulmonary embolus, a wound infection and a three week hospitalization.

My first exposure to the existence of this entity came on a snowy February day at a Catholic teaching hospital in Boston. Sister Flaherty**, the operating room supervisor, came into the operating theater. She noted the progress of the case, looked at the attending surgeon and said, in a perfect Barry Fitzgerald Bells of St. Mary's Irish brogue: "I don't mean to give you the k'enohorah Dr. Felfman, but I see that this case went very well!"

Surgery is both art and science. The science is pretty straightforward. The art influences the discipline in many ways, some of which border on the mystical.

The surgical k'enohorah is one of those mystical influences.

** Not her real name.

Matrix Lesson 31

All laparoscopic cables and tubing become intertwined, despite any attempt at logical arrangement

---

The Laparoscopic Revolution forever changed the face of general surgery. Its introduction has caused surgeons to re-orient their view of operative surgery. To a degree, all working general surgeons must now be basic physicists. Many great physicists have contributed to the field of laparoscopic surgery. One of the greatest contributions was by Renée Descarte. Matrix Lesson 31 is based on the pioneering work of this brilliant physicist.

A mathematician and philosopher (he could add and, at the same time think about why he was adding), Descarte contributed greatly to an understanding of laparoscopic physics. His theory of vortices accounts for many explanations in today's operating rooms. His "Rational Basis for Hypothesis of Creation of the Solar System" explains many of our laparoscopic light source problems.

But it is for his Vortex Theory that he is remembered most by surgeons. Studying the logic theory of tube placement, he became fascinated by the evolving randomness of a concerted non-random action. He initially studied the placement of tubes in the laboratory. Eventually he became hospital-based and geographically full-time. Subsequently, he became operating room-based. Reducing tube and wire placement to a mathematical equation occupied his later years.

"Hitherto neatly operative fields are now coiled affairs with flowing fluids, electrical cables and gas lines."

This burgeoning discipline of studying tubes and cords is at the heart of laparoscopic surgery. Hitherto neatly operative fields are now coiled affairs with flowing fluids, electrical cables and gas lines. Descartes anticipated this arrangement and decided that it needed to be formulated into a mathematical model.

Just prior to his death, he wrote his Vortex Theory in German, *Die Tuben Verschimmelt*, in which he states his theory that all laparoscopic cables and tubes become randomly intertwined, despite the surgeon's efforts to straighten them out.

I have translated *Die Tuben Verschimmelt* and present it to the working laparoscopist as Matrix Lesson #31.

Adapted from: Gordon LA. The Physics of Laparoscopic Surgery: A Dissertation on the Contributions of Famous Physicists to Laparoscopic Surgery. *Perspectives in Biology and Medicine* 1997; 40(4).

Matrix Lesson 32

The case scheduled for three

hours will take one hour

"Obverse of Matrix Lesson #32: the case scheduled for one hour will take three hours."

A resident presenting at the Matrix Conference is frequently asked the duration of the case being discussed. I have never been sold on the concept that the fastest surgeon is the better surgeon or that the slower surgeon is somehow less gifted or expert.

What governs the length of a surgical case is a weird, wonderful and ultimately inexplicable force. Every experienced surgeon, office manager and operating room administrator understands Matrix Lesson #32.

Surgery is a discipline of anatomic discovery. That process of discovery evolves during the operation. To date there is no scan, test or film that can show the same things the surgeon sees and feels during his operation.

The slam-dunk laparoscopic cholecystectomy in a thin twenty-nine year-old will turn out to have acute cholecystitis and a ductal anomaly. The elective resection for diverticulitis will turn out to have a confined perforation involving the ureter.

These events prove on a daily basis that the essence of general surgery is a set of anatomic challenges, not a rote repetition of hand motions and decision algorithms. Why then, are a certain number of nurses and colleagues surprised when surgical cases take longer than the time requested?

The reasons are varied but usually have to do with some unfounded perception that the surgical day can actually be co-ordinated and that human pathology can be made, by administrative feat, to conform to someone's wishes. The case which runs longer than expected, because of an unexpected or difficult finding, is the surgical gods' way of saying that *they are still and always will be in control.*

We have a small sign hung in our office waiting room which states that "delays in the operative schedule, cases which take longer than expected and emergency situations may prevent our surgeons from being on time for your office visit. Your understanding is appreciated."

"These events prove on a daily basis that the essence of general surgery is a set of anatomic challenges, not a rote repetition of hand motions and decision algorithms."

I'm not sure anyone reads this sign or pays attention to it. It is a feeble attempt to explain to patients what happens in an operating room.

I am always amazed when my colleagues do not understand this, as their cases are delayed. Angry surgeons whose case follows in the room, dismayed office managers, and perskinnity operating room co-ordinators continually poke their respective noses in the room, mystified and dumbfounded when Matrix Lesson #32 kicks in. Their inability to grasp this fact of surgical life is a testament to their lack of appreciation for the essence of surgery.

Happily, Lesson #32 has an obverse. Occasionally, the "cement abdomen," the "infiltrating tumor" and the "encased vessels" will be merely radiological ephemera and will present no problem to the surgeon. Such anatomic vagaries are usually attributed to superior surgical skills. The three hours blocked out, magically, has the surgeon drinking coffee in ninety minutes.

The surgical gods have smiled on that particular day.

Matrix Lesson 33

No-one knows the proper nomenclature
for the ligaments of the spleen

The greatest semantic surgical tragedy is the retention of the Latin root for the word spleen. This root (*lien*) is used to name the ligaments of the spleen. The ancient anatomists did not know the horror and confusion they would create by doing this.

The fact that it rhymes with spleen and is alliterative with the prefix ren- for kidney, created inextricably difficult rhyming ligamentous confusion.

When anatomy was fifty percent of the medical school curriculum there were probably two or three weeks spent on naming these ligaments. Since that curriculum now is crowded with more important courses, the time spent on anatomy is less. Because of this, the specific naming of the ligaments of the spleen has lessened in importance.

Take the following quiz:

Which of the following are ligamentous attachments of the spleen?

- The lieno-reno.
- The Janet Reno.
- The reno-lieno.
- The spleeno-reno.
- The Reno-bambino (in pediatric surgery).
- The lieno-spleeno.
- The Valentino-reno-spleeno (the ligament joining a ruptured spleen to a perforated ulcer).
- The spleeno-lieno-reno.
- The spleeno-maraschino (the ligament joining the spleen to the lead point of a small bowel obstruction caused by a cherry pit).
- The lieno-reno-spleeno.
- The Harrah's Tahoe Reno (also known as the casino-Reno).
- The spleeno-palomino (taught only in veterinary school).

One can see the difficulties here.

In fact, *no-one* knows the correct names of these ligaments.

I feel great joy when I walk into an operating room and hear various prominent attending surgeons demonstrating and explaining these splenic ligaments to unsuspecting surgical residents. The dialogue, or monologue, in most cases, goes like this: "Yes. Here is the reno-spleeno ligament. That there is the lieno-reno ligament. Oh, quick, watch, I just cut the beano-spleeno-reno ligament."

How residents control their laughter is beyond me.

"In fact, no-one knows the correct names of these ligaments."

If you are asked on your surgical board examinations by the examiner: "Describe the ligamentous attachments of the spleen." Your answer should be: [Inhale deeply as if going underwater, then blurt out] "The lieno-reno, the spleeno-eno, the lieno-reno-beano - the beano-lieno-Janet Reno, the Reno-maraschino and the spleeno-beano-reno."

When enunciated clearly and with the proper professorial cadence, one is assured a passing grade.

Matrix Lesson 34

If the gynecologist says it is not adnexal, it is *always* adnexal

A frequent topic of discussion at the Matrix Conference is the "error in diagnosis." Prior to the advent of the CT scan and sophisticated sonography, a common error was operating on a patient presumed to have appendicitis who, in fact, had adnexal disease.

Differentiating the signs and symptoms of appendicitis from adnexal pathology is the key to an accurate diagnosis. The signs and symptoms of these two disorders may overlap. On careful interview and examination, however, these two disease entities could be differentiated. This effort was often collaborative between the general surgeon and the gynecologist.

It is illogical to consider appendicitis as the primary diagnosis when a menstruating mid-cycle female with the sudden onset of right lower quadrant pain and a robust appetite presents to the emergency department. Fluid in the *cul-de-sac* on an ultrasound usually makes the diagnosis of an adnexal problem.

"But for some inexplicable reason many gynecologists cannot recognize the clinical pattern of a ruptured ovarian cyst without the involvement of a general surgeon."

Which leads us to a consideration of one of the more mystifying aspects of the discipline of gynecology. This principle states: summon a general surgeon for all but the most obvious of pelvic emergencies to shoulder the responsibility of assessing, defining and treating that emergency. To do so, state, with a straight face, that the adnexal disease is actually not adnexal. In other words - if it is adnexal, say it is not adnexal.

I respect my gynecologic colleagues. They perform a great medical service whenever they lyse filmy peritubular adhesions. They can chart when the FSH rises, the LH plunges and the HCG levels off. They can perform version and can wax eloquent on double footling breeches. In addition to this, it must never be forgotten that it was the gynecologists who stumbled onto the critical role of the light source in the performance of safe operative laparoscopy.

But for some inexplicable reason many gynecologists cannot recognize the clinical pattern of a ruptured ovarian cyst *without the involvement of a general surgeon*. It is as if they have an extra lobe in their brain - a lobe in which resides the genetic compulsion to transfer care to a general surgeon.

This cerebral zone, located deep within the rhinencephalon of the gynecologist is the "general surgical displacement zone." Autopsy studies have shown that this area, refined over the millenia of gynecologic activity, causes the gynecologist to displace the responsibility for diagnosis and treatment onto another consultant, usually the general surgeon. Archaeological studies have revealed that the Ur-gynecologist, a well-meaning Cro-magnon, got into the habit of placing wounded tribe members into the cave of a neighbor. He then retreated into the mists of the plain, leaving the care and comfort of the wounded party to that neighbor. Within the general surgical displacement zone, the gynecologic cerebral circuitry is so wired that analytic thought frequently veers away from the gynecologically logical, the gynecologically plausible and the gynecologically common-sensical. We have a displacement of intellect and a displacement of responsibility.

Every gynecologist has this area within his or her brain. This is the physiologic explanation for the otherwise inexplicable tendency to arrive at consistently wrong conclusions about adnexal disease. The general surgical displacement zone explains why, when a gynecologist is summoned to the general surgical operating theater to view an inflamed tube oozing pus he will look at the team and state: "See, I told you it's not adnexal!"

It is now 03:35 hrs. on a warm California summer night. I am in the emergency room evaluating a twenty-nine-year-old woman with the sudden onset of right lower quadrant pain. I am speaking to the consultant gynecologist who, of course, said it was not adnexal.

In a flash of surgical candor, I say that he had just fulfilled the basic tenet of Matrix Lesson #34. He asked what I meant. I replied: "If the gynecologist said it is not adnexal, it is always adnexal." The reaction is predictable. I am dismissed from the care of the patient.

Matrix Lesson 35

A prepared presentation never gets presented

> "Obverse of Law #35: a presentation which is not prepared always gets presented."

Matrix Lesson #35 is for the residents.

It is axiomatic that the harder a resident works on a presentation, the less likely it is that that presentation will ever be presented.

For example, a resident is rounding with Professor A. The resident is anxious to impress Professor A for several reasons. Professor A is on the Resident Evaluation Committee. Professor A will be the resident's attending next month. Frankly, Professor A has complete control over the resident's happiness and existence. Rounds are underway. Internal hernias are mentioned during a case presentation of a patient with a small bowel obstruction. As is his wont, Professor A looks at the resident and says: "You know, a brief presentation on the history and surgical approaches to internal hernias would be very welcome next week on rounds." A light goes off in the resident's brain - "I will prepare this presentation. I will do it for the purity of surgical education, but even tactically more rewarding, I will do it to fulfill the very high expectations Professor A has for me." Rounds end.

"The educational benefit is in the preparation, not the presentation."

The metaphysical basis of Lesson #35 follows. The resident is involved in many emergencies. He is sleepless, driven, and exhausted. And yet, from the depths of his being, drawing on his last remaining powers, he schleps himself to the library and prepares a presentation on internal intestinal herniation. He takes notes. He Xeroxes. He powerpoints and prepares handouts. He immerses himself in the embryology of the foregut and the hindgut. He researches Winslow and his foramen. He translates from the original German "Die Kishkes Ungestoppt." He, has, in fact, committed the cardinal error of a surgical residency - he has taken the Professor seriously!

Rounds with Professor A approach. The resident is ready. He is confident. He is ..... forgotten! Know this and know this well: the presentation so skillfully prepared will *never* be presented. The Professor has totally forgotten about it! An emergency will occur. The presenting resident will be called to the emergency room or, for purely academic reasons (an open handball court), the Professor will cancel the rounds. The prepared presentation is never presented.

The benefit of presenting anything, whether it is a brief historical vignette of Frau Heller, Billroth's first gastrectomy, or grand rounds at a major medical center, effects only one person - the resident who had to prepare it. The educational benefit is in the preparation, not the presentation. That is as it should be, since a prepared presentation never gets presented.

Now on to one of the trickier aspects of resident life. A presentation which has not been prepared, is always presented.

Here is where skillful resident activity is so important. The resident has gambled and has lost. It is essential at this point to have what is called a resident ally. Upon hearing the call for the presentation, the resident ally shrewdly clutches his beeper, retreats to a wall phone and .... pages the presenting resident in an urgent manner.

His beeper repeatedly beeps. Feigning annoyance at being interrupted, the presenting resident looks at Professor A and says: "Excuse me, I have to answer this page ..."

He returns to the assemblage, looks at Professor A and says: "I'm sorry, that was Dr. X (substitute the name of the chief of surgery). He wants to see me right away!"

A brief digression into the world of surgical academia is in order. The chief holds the career promises for Professor A just as Professor A governs the daily existence of the presenting resident. It is nothing more than the daily activity of the academic food-chain.

For that reason Professor A yields to the call of his superior. Academic stratification has been recognized. The resident saves face and Professor A can go on to make more inane presentation assignments.

It is best to have some form of preparation ready, but also to have a fall-back position as outlined above. Surgical education is a very personal endeavor of which preparation for seminars and presentations is quite important. Matrix Lesson #35 puts that endeavor into perspective.

Matrix Lesson 36

Never violate Occam's Razor

I referred to William of Occam in Matrix Lesson #21. His principles and philosophy are so important to surgery, that they require their own recognition and their own Matrix Lesson. The lesson relies on streamlined surgical logic - the essence of expeditious and accurate surgical diagnosis.

William of Occam was a philosopher who lived in the early 1500s. He liked to argue the fine points of an issue. It was as if he dissected every argument with a razor.

In those days trademark names were all the vogue - The Great, The Unready, the Conqueror, the Razor, etc. I tried to revive this vogue at my own hospital, but individual colleagues did not like the appellation "Phil the Abscess Causer", or "Sid the Embolus King." Anyhow,

William of Occam encouraged the principle that things do not have to be proven beyond the point of their proof. As he stated it: *Entia non sunt miltiplicanda praeter necessitatem.* Entities are not to be multiplied beyond need.

Occam used this principle as a powerful tool of logic "cutting away a hundred occult fancies and grandiose abstractions."* Putting Occam's philosophy into a medical context means that the proof of disease need not be unnecessarily duplicated. Or put in a Freudian context - sometimes a hot dog is just a hot dog! Or, as my uncle Lou might say: "Don't beat me over the head with it."

Experienced practical surgeons have used Occam's Razor for many years. It separates the surgeons from the philosophers, who are often lost in a morass of ever escalating duplicatory proofs of common diseases.

The penchant for the surgical mind to follow Occam's Razor is the reason that many people feel that if all patients were admitted to the surgical service, medical care in this country would be more efficient.

"Putting Occam's philosophy into a medical context means that the proof of disease need not be unnecessarily duplicated."

Eloquently stated by Mark Ravitch in his editorial "An Opportunity to Lower Costs and Elevate the Quality of Medical Care,"** this idea has more merit than any Washington focus-group could ever formulate.

* *The Story of Civilization.* Vol. VI. *The Reformation.* Will Durant. New York: MJF Books, 1957: 246-7.
** Ravitch MM. An Opportunity to Lower Costs and Elevate the Quality of Medical Care. *Surgical Rounds* 1982; March: 8-9.

Ravitch's plan is stated in two pages. It is precise, clear and logical. A certain First Lady's proposal for healthcare ran 1156 pages. It was muddled, illogical and, in the end, laughable.

William of Occam should be the Secretary of Health and Human Services. But that's for the next administration. Violating Occam's Razor is expensive. It subjects the patient to unnecessary risks and delays in treatment.

Here are some representative Razor violations:

- A fifty-two-year-old male with a history of ulcer disease comes to the emergency room with a rigid abdomen and free air under the diaphragm.
  A water soluble contrast swallow is ordered.
- An eighteen-year-old female presents with mid-cycle pain and right lower quadrant tenderness.
  A gastrograffin enema, ultrasound and culdocentesis are ordered.
- A sixty-eight-year-old male with a history of gallstones presents with a globular right upper quadrant mass, fever and jaundice.
  A CAT scan, HIDA scan, ERCP and transhepatic cholangiogram are ordered.
- A seventy-five-year-old male presents with an asymptomatic low output cecal fistula after an appendectomy.
  A sinogram, barium enema and upper gastrointestinal series are ordered.
- An eighty-three-year-old male with a pulsatile abdominal mass presents urgently with back pain, shock and anemia.
  A CT scan and angiogram are ordered.

Occam's Razor is a valuable surgical reasoning tool. Matrix Lesson #36 reminds us to use it as we analyze surgical problems.

Matrix Lesson 37

If the nurses like you, you are not doing your job

Nurses are essential to the smooth and effective administration of a surgical service. Over the years, they have ascended in importance to the point where, as of this writing, an experienced surgical nurse is probably in greater demand than an experienced surgeon.

Want ads in major metropolitan dailies are not seeking an "earnest surgical resident with Ivy League education and eye on advancement." They are crying for nurses. Nurses can go to any city in this country, find a job with high pay and good benefits, and can then write their own tickets.

The relationship between surgeons and nurses has always been a particularly delicate one. Relating to nurses in a co-operative and mutually beneficial manner has always been a challenge for the surgeon.

This fact was first pointed out by no less prominent a surgeon than Epectetus, during the construction of his surgicenter on Thrace. He imported Peloponessian nurses to staff his operating theater. It was from that association that the relationship between surgeons and nurses grew.

Surgeons demand a lot of themselves, and for that reason demand a lot from nurses and operating room personnel. It is contradictory and illogical to demand something from a person and then balance that demand with an overwhelming desire to be liked or admired. These demands and these desires are, as the French might say, at contretemps.

"It is impossible to deliver the highest quality of surgical care without demanding a great deal from the nursing staff."

If the surgeon's prime goal is satisfaction of the nursing staff over and above patient care considerations, he is off the mark. He is liked, but he is a surgical failure. The nurses cannot perform up to the highest standards, any more than a surgeon himself can perform to the highest standards, *unless challenged on a daily basis*. Part of that challenge for nurses is working with surgeons who demand perfection in patient care.

There are surgeons whose goal is to be the "nice guy" or the "nurse's friend." Perhaps their wives are rough on them. Perhaps they were never chosen for the softball team in high school. Whatever it was, now its thirty years later and they feel compelled not to criticize a nurse who: has taken off the wrong order; or, does not know what operation the patient had undergone. These surgeons are weak links in the surgical chain of perfection.

It seems to be a sad fact of the medical workplace that the less anyone demands of a worker, the better that person is liked. Matrix Lesson #37 follows.

Observe this anomaly on your own surgical wards. The demanding surgeons appear - the nurses run for cover. The smarm-meisters appear - it is as if a rock star entered.

It is impossible to deliver the highest quality of surgical care without demanding a great deal from the nursing staff.

It is proper for surgeons to demand a lot from the nurses. The nurses will not like you, but they sure will pay more attention to you. In so doing they will take better care of the patients.

Matrix Lesson 38

Leave your attitude outside
of the operating theater

My children used to go to summer camp in the Texas hill country outside of San Antonio. A lot has happened to summer camps since I went to Camp Lawrence on Lake Winnepesaukee in New Hampshire (eight weeks, $240 in 1959). Now children have to take a jet and a camp limousine to partake in recreational psychosocial development in a non-threatening, environmentally conscious, peer-structured summer residential enrichment program to foster multicultural awareness in a gender-neutral religion-free environment. But that's for another book.

One summer, we dropped our children off and then went out for an authentic hill country Texas dinner. Amazingly, on the menu were no free range chicken, arugula or shitake mushrooms. We found just what we were looking for - charred slabs of beef, potatoes and bread. We were seated near the bar. Over the bar was a yellowed framed sign which stated: "Leave your attitude outside."

"... don't get an attitude."

Any observer of the bar scene knew exactly what it meant. The bar is a place for quiet recreation and contemplation - a place with a uniform goal for all of its patrons - enjoyment. The operating theater, although unable to deliver a passable martini, has a similar aura and a similar goal.

The people in the OR, especially the operating surgeon, are there for one reason - to perform the surgery as effectively as possible. Professional enjoyment flows from this precept.

Everything else in the operating theater is secondary to that goal. And yet, many people other than the surgeon are in the operating room - the scrub nurse, the anesthesiologist, the circulating nurse, the resident. Each has his own day, his own set of priorities, and his own set of problems. Occasionally, those problems can intrude onto the flow of the case.

The surgeon himself may, as I stated to my children when they were younger, have been visited by Mr. Grumpy. He may bring his daily baggage into the operating theater. The nurse may dislike the surgeon, or may have other problems. She may bring her baggage into the operating theater. The resident's student loan payment may be in arrears. He may be concerned about it. His girlfriend may have dismissed him because of his schedule. The anesthesiologist's tax shelter may have been disallowed by the Internal Revenue Service. Each of these situations has its own attitude.

A semantic digression is in order. The term "don't get an attitude" requires an explanation. When I was growing up the word *attitude* meant one of three things. It meant the placement of a figure in a painting. What is the attitude of the lead figure in Breugel's "The Blind

Leading the Blind?" Or it meant the orientation of something as it was traveling. What was the *attitude* of the airplane as it descended? Finally, it meant an opinion or point of view, i.e. "What is your attitude towards socialized medicine."

Over the last several years, attitude has taken on a new meaning - a set of beliefs or a demeanor that is distasteful or unruly, such as is used in the phrases "Lose the attitude!" or "Drop the attitude." This is the meaning as stated on the sign in the bar in Texas. This is the theme of Matrix Lesson #38.

The attitudes of the people mentioned above can find their way into the operating theater. Political attitudes, personal attitudes, attitudes regarding hospital policies, or even attitudes towards various surgical procedures can be voiced.

There is always a place for discussion in the operating theater. Occasionally, there is even a place for spirited debate over surgical principle. But there is no room for attitude, in the currently defined sense of the word.

As the snippety, the obnoxious or the counter-productive approach the operating theater, Matrix Lesson #38 is quite clear - leave your attitude outside the operating theater!

Matrix Lesson 39

Cancel this case!

I never park in space #13 or #113 in the physicians' parking lot. I never play blackjack at a table with a dealer whose first name begins with "L." I never board a plane before knocking twice on the fuselage. I never watch a Red Sox game unless my father's 1973 copy of *What's the Matter with the Red Sox?* is by my side.*

Which is *why I never* proceed with a case if there is any intimation that things are not just right.

Some examples:

- A 69-year-old executive arrives for an outpatient hernia repair. He is seen in the pre-operative holding area where he states to the surgeon: "Things don't seem right."

* Hirshberg A. *What's the Matter with the Red Sox?* New York: Dodd, Mead & Co., 1973.

- A 28-year-old female arrives on the 15th of the month for a laparoscopic cholecystectomy. She states: "You know, fifteen has always been an unlucky number for me."
- An 83-year-old male with a colon lesion arrives for a colectomy after a bowel prep. He states: "I had some cramping in my chest on the way in this morning."
- An otherwise healthy 59-year-old male arrives for excision of a melanoma and a groin dissection. A pre-operative EKG is read by the computer as "abnormal." A call is made to the patient's internist who states: "It's been like that for years."

"The surgical gods are telling you something."

There is no science, no "evidence-based" surgical fact, no "outcome data" or double-blind study to support what I am about to say, but hear me and hear me well: *cancel this case!* You may have an angry patient. You may lose a referral. You may invoke the ire of the scheduling people, your office staff, or even your colleagues. The surgical gods are telling you something. They are giving you a warning - something very rare for the operating surgeon.

Oh, I can feel the groans now floating onto this page. But ... the patient had to take a day off of work. But ... the internist said there were no changes on the EKG. But ... you really don't believe in that astrological-numerological mumbo-jumbo do you? Hear this and hear this well: there are mysterious forces at work in our profession. Sometimes they will show their hand in the subtlest of ways. Listen for them. Look for them. And when you hear or see them, heed their warnings.

Cancel the case!

Matrix
Lesson 40

Anticipation is the single greatest
attribute of a premier scrub nurse

When I glance at the back table and see the proper
sutures and instruments prepared for my case ... when I
look at the nurse's most readily accessible instruments
and they are perched neatly on a folded green towel ....
when the nurse hands me the proper instrument of the
proper length at the proper time for the proper portion of
the operation .... when the flawless cadence of a truly
prepared operating room nurse is rhythmically
synchronized with my own motions ... when the length of
suture is consistent with the depth of the field ... when the
light source is plugged in ... when it really seems that, in
fact, this is not the first low anterior resection ever
performed on the West Coast ... or when it seems that, in
fact, it is not 1890 and the concept of a gastrectomy is
not an abstract theory by an Austrian surgeon, but a
daily event ... then I know that the nurse is not only
prepared, but that she or he *anticipates* the surgeon's

move. Anticipation is the single greatest attribute of the premier scrub nurse.

"... the truly great nurse will know that surgeon and will anticipate his moves."

Operations fall into predictable patterns, yet only a minority of scrub nurses seem to get a professional handle on that pattern. Although surgeons differ in preference, speed and talent, the truly great nurse will know that surgeon and will anticipate his moves.

After long and serious study (not controlled, not double-blind and quite random), I have come to the conclusion that this skill of operative anticipation cannot be taught.

It is a personal trait, not a nursing trait. It is a trait built into the psyche of those who wish to propel themselves to the top of their fields. It is the same trait that allowed Larry Bird to pass the ball not to where his teammate was, but to where he would be. It is a valuable trait - the single most valuable trait of an excellent nurse. It marks her with the same professional traits that make some surgeons excellent surgeons - anticipation.

When the scrub nurse anticipates the needs of the case and of the surgeon, all is right with the surgical world.

Matrix Lesson 41

The emergency room is the best
place to evaluate an emergency

Emergency rooms were designed for the expeditious care of ill patients. Inpatient hospital ward beds and doctors' offices were not.

This concept is foreign to many physicians. These physicians have a concept called the "direct admission." It is a rather unique approach to the orderly and efficient workup of common medical and surgical problems.

The philosophy behind the "direct admission" is the belief that an urgent problem is best evaluated once the patient is ensconced in a bed on an inpatient ward. It is a lot like saying: "I have a ruptured aneurysm!" and having the next logical thought be: "I must check in to the Holiday Inn and request the room furthest away from the desk!"

The *worst* place to evaluate an emergency admission is on a patient ward. The circumstance is urgent. The surroundings are totally elective. These conditions are at loggerheads.

I get many calls from internists about emergencies (this will not be the case after publication of this book). Invariably, the conversation ends, with "... and I've arranged a direct admission." I call this the Direct Emergency Admission Time Hurdle (D.E.A.T.H.), since the time to obtain the most basic of studies to evaluate an urgent complaint is prolonged by the ward location of the patient.

My office staff became very expert at intercepting patients throughout Los Angeles and guiding them to various emergency rooms.

On an inpatient floor the lab work, the X-rays, and other studies are always tough to organize and to obtain. The mindset of the floor personnel is different from the mindset of the emergency room personnel. The average "direct admission" sets the average physician back about one to two hours over an emergency room evaluation.

"The worst place to evaluate an emergency admission is on a patient ward."

Economic factors notwithstanding, the emergency room is the best place for the evaluation of new problems. With its centralized laboratory and X-ray facilities, it is ideal for urgent evaluations. One can get to the operating theater more quickly, assemble the lab data and generally firm up a diagnosis in a more fluid manner.

Matrix Lesson #41 encourages you to diplomatically and skillfully channel emergent referrals to the emergency room.

Matrix
Lesson 42

Never discuss your pension plan

Today's residents are more economically savvy than at any other time in the history of medicine. They should be.

They went through medical school during the greatest economic analysis of medicine in the history of the world. Healthcare reform and debate formed the background of their medical development. They owe money for student loans and are concerned about making a living in the future. Many of the residents have investments and various pension plans. This notwithstanding, the discussion of personal economic issues has no place on the ward or in the operating theater.

In particular, the attending surgeon should never discuss his pension plan. What is this plan? It is a sum of money that the government allows you to set aside and invest for your retirement years. It is not taxed. If properly managed, it grows (unless you follow the advice of a certain broker from a certain prominent brokerage house who tells you to invest a certain percentage of your money in a certain biotech company whose fortunes happen to end up as certain worthless stock certificates!).

"Create a pension plan. Contribute to the pension plan. Manage the pension plan. But never discuss your pension plan!"

What most surgeons do not realize about their plans is that they will never live to enjoy one penny of it. They will be dead!

The most over-riding reason to never discuss a pension plan is illustrated by the following vignette. This scenario is most poignantly recalled when you are in the emergency room at 3AM draining a buttock abscess:

Here it is. You are dead. Hopefully, you are in surgical heaven where the cases start on time. Raoul, the pony-tailed waiter from Le Peregrine, is lying on a chaise lounge on the beach in Grand Cayman Island. The sky is cloudless. The water is cerulescent. Raoul is young. He is tanned. He is thin. Each of his oiled (SPF 35), tendinous inscriptions shines in the Caribbean sun. He is drinking one of those drinks with a small paper parasol in it. He is wearing a lycra bathing suit that is essentially a marble bag. In short, Raoul is your wife's fantasy-man. The man who is everything you were not. She is lying next to him. Raoul calls for a cabana boy. His drink arrives. He sips it. He frowns. He is disappointed with the drink. He sends the drink back because it does not have the proper amount of anastago bitters. The cabana boy returns. Raoul gives him a generous tip. That tip is your pension money!

Create a pension plan. Contribute to the pension plan. Manage the pension plan. But never *discuss* your pension plan!

Matrix Lesson 43

Never discuss the asymptomatic
carotid bruit

We are all familiar with certain social situations in which topics are bought up which we, for a variety of reasons, do not want to discuss. Perhaps it relates to a former partner, or a nasty malpractice suit. Perhaps your son's arraignment found its way onto the local news section. Whatever it is, we shy away from such topics because they are inextricably difficult to bow out of graciously.

I feel that way about vascular surgery in general and about the asymptomatic carotid bruit in particular. My deep resentment towards vascular surgery (the first and most successful marketing ploy in American surgery) is based on its total disregard for the gastrointestinal tract. The entire gastrointestinal system to vascular surgeons is an incidental finding on the way to the aorta!

This active digestive tube ... this marvelous conduit that can handle a breakfast burrito or veal marsala ... this supremely democratic flesh tube that has no regard for its content's station in life ... this egalitarian energizer that puts a chili dog on equal footing with the veal patenouf with shitake mushrooms ... this England! But I digress!

Vascular surgeons toss aside the gastrointestinal tract, pack it, retract it and generally disregard it, as they go about their business. Vascular surgery seems to suit people with a solid manual arts background rather than a medical background.

This flippant action is a direct affront to me and to all that I hold dear. It is the seed of my dislike for this general surgical stepchild. Adding to this underlying feeling is the most specious topic in all of vascular surgery - the discussion of the management and controversies surrounding the asymptomatic carotid bruit.

The management of the asymptomatic carotid bruit is not a medical problem; it is a philosophical problem. Why else would every journal of vascular surgery have fifteen papers about this entity? Every month - papers, seminars, controversies, arguments, debates, cruises, junkets, retreats, focus groups, break-out sessions, congresses, conclaves, meetings - enough already!

> "It would seem to me that for medical and environmental reasons, noisy arteries should be cleaned out."

The professoriate has, by design and custom, made the problem inextricably difficult. The problem is really quite simple - God gave us two pipes to perfuse our brain. Because of chili rejeño, veal piccata and the cheese blintz, these pipes get clogged. When they get clogged particles build up and cause a noise. The significance of this noise is the central point of the arguments and discussions.

On and on it goes - aspirin, coumadin, surgery, stenting - on and on, forever and ever, in an ever widening spiral of papers, research projects, double-blind studies, triple-blind studies and consensus reports.

What to do with this noise? If you are awake and alert and know your artery is making a noise, it should be fixed. If you are confused and cannot think clearly and someone points out that the artery is making a noise, it should be fixed. Either way - it should be fixed. It is noisy. It is annoying.

Do you want, as my dear departed father would say, to "take a stroke?" (My Dad always thought people *took* their illnesses - he took a heart attack. He took a stroke. It is as if life gives you a smorgasbord of disease from which to choose. Oh me? I'll have the aneurysm with a side of aphasia thank you!).

It would seem to me that for medical and environmental reasons, noisy arteries should be cleaned out. The benefits are obvious - less stress on the ozone layer by noise pollution, clearer thinking by people and generally better cerebral perfusion. These are lofty goals which should prevent the asymptomatic carotid bruit from ever being discussed again in proper company.

It is telling that one of the literal translations of the French word *bruit* is "rumor." Perhaps the French linguists anticipated the day when professors of vascular surgery would start a rumor that weighty and meaningful controversy existed in their discipline - the management of the asymptomatic carotid bruit.

Matrix Lesson 44

Never refuse 07:30 Hrs. operating time

Some surgeons do not accept 07:30 Hrs. operating time. Maybe they are exercising. Maybe they like to sleep late. Maybe they have lost touch with their surgical roots.

There are two reasons for accepting 07:30 Hrs. operating time and for making it a guiding principle never to refuse such time when it is offered. The first reason is quite simple - the surgical day is impossible to arrange.

It behooves the working surgeon to get his cases done as early in the day as possible. Seven-thirty cases have an excellent chance of starting on time. It is unlikely that they will be delayed due to emergencies. Seven-thirty time allows the surgeon to become an expert in "clock management," a guiding principle of other professional teams, most notably football after the two-minute warning.

The second and more important reason for never refusing seven-thirty time is a spiritual reason. To appreciate this spirituality one must view the row of scrub sinks at any hospital just before seven-thirty.

> "Seven-thirty time allows the surgeon to become an expert in 'clock management.'"

Surgeons are scrubbing, nurses are preparing - the day is a clean slate. The scene is a heroic metaphor for anticipated success. It is like the fifteen minutes before a prize-fight or the time just before a playoff game. The promise of a spectacular day is there. All of the hopes, all of the aspirations, all of the goals of clinical surgery are just waiting to be achieved and realized.

Nothing has happened yet. The case lies ahead. One cannot get this feeling at any other time in the surgical day. It is an exhilarating feeling. It is a daily renewal of surgical enthusiasm.

If one could bottle the essence of the fifteen minutes before these morning cases, one would have the essence of pride in one's work and the essence of the determination to see that that work is done expertly.

This is the best reason for *always* accepting seven-thirty surgery time.

Matrix
Lesson 45

Call patients facing outpatient surgery the
night before surgery and the night of surgery

Mr. Herbert Rose*, a short New Jersey accountant, sat down with a legal pad and several No. 2 pencils in 1983 and figured out that the famous and traditional "night before surgery" admission cost the country about 2 billion dollars a year.

Because of Mr. Rose, insurance companies began to deny payment to hospitals for "night before surgery" admissions. This was good accounting and good cost-containment, but it destroyed a great and honored aspect of medicine - the night before surgery visit.

Some older readers may remember the "night before surgery" admission. After the day's surgery and after the office, a surgeon would make evening rounds. He would see some of his postoperative patients.

* Herbert Rose is not his real name. His real name is Sidney Rose.

Then he would see patients preparing for surgery for the next day - patients who had been admitted that afternoon in preparation for surgery. The surgeon would sit down next to the bed and go over the points made in the office visit. The patient would be confident that the surgeon remembered the office visit. The surgeon would be confident that he remembered the particular points of the patient's history and physical examination. Questions would be answered. Fears and concerns would be addressed. This "night before surgery" meeting was a wonderful part of medicine - for the patient and for the surgeon. Herbert Rose eliminated it. We now have the concept of the AM admission.

"Just as pre-operative phone calls allay pre-operative fears, so do postoperative phone calls allay postoperative concerns."

Instead of rested and calm pre-operative patients, we now have characters in the middle of a Kafka novel. Waking up at five AM, delivered in the gray dawn to a faceless institution, facing surgery with fear, apprehension and annoyance, patients are herded to the operating theater. Contrast this to the patient rested and at peace because of a pre-operative hospital visit by his surgeon.

What can the surgeon do to counter-balance this situation? What can he do to retrieve some of the benefit of the night before surgery visit? We cannot sit at the bedside before surgery, but we can call the patient the night before surgery.

The phone is impersonal. It lacks eye contact. It cannot provide a warm touch or a confident demeanor. One cannot re-examine a patient telephonically (although some older surgeons will disagree with this). Nevertheless, the phone call is effective. It establishes the immediate pre-operative patient-surgeon bond that the face-to-face visit used to establish. Most of these pre-operative conversations end with a heartfelt, "Thanks for calling," allaying some of the pre-operative fears.

Similarly, we no longer can examine and converse with many postoperative patients. They are at home icing their scrota after hernia repairs. Just as pre-operative phone calls allay pre-operative fears, so do postoperative phone calls allay postoperative concerns.

Call outpatients before and after surgery. It is a poor substitute for the classical surgical face-to-face visit, but is greatly appreciated by all patients.

Matrix Lesson 46

The attending physician is always right

Matrix Lesson #46 will save residents a lot of time and wasted energy. It is a blackletter medical law.

I must codify this most basic principle of the surgical hierarchy. Notice the wording of the law. It does not say the "professor" is always right. It says the *attending* is *always* right. It is the motto of the successful surgical resident.

The attending surgeon has been through his education program. The attending surgeon has taken his board examinations. The attending surgeon has weathered the storm of clinical practice. The attending surgeon has been on the Medical Records Committee. The attending surgeon has attended the chief's Christmas party. In short, the attending surgeon has paid his surgical dues.

While honest differences of opinion regarding management and surgical practice do arise on any service, the resident must, as the song goes, "know when to hold them and know when to fold them." That's why Lesson #46 was formulated - to provide stability and form to the surgical service.

"... the law ... It says the attending is always right. It is the motto of the successful surgical resident."

It behooves the resident to know when to surrender, unless of course, it is a critical issue likely to injure a patient. In these situations, fortunately infrequent, Article 1 of Lesson #46 (attending error) may be invoked. This needs a two-thirds majority by the entire medical staff and is somewhat difficult to organize.

Residents who follow this Matrix Lesson #46 are assured of excellent resident evaluations, glowing letters of recommendation and perhaps a future partnership position.

There is a reason for this lesson. It provides order. It provides framework and structure to the surgical service.

Matrix
Lesson 47

The quality of the X-ray ordered is directly proportional to the specificity of the clinical information supplied to the radiologist

$$Q = x/p$$
Q = quality of the study
x = amount of clinical information supplied
p = pathology suspected.

At the top of most radiology* requisition slips is the term "radiologic consultation." It does not usually say "X-ray request." It does not say "lab test."

It says it is a consultation. Just as a surgeon would provide needed data to a cardiologic consultant, an infectious disease consultant or a neurological consultant, so must that information be provided to the radiologic consultant.

* "Radiologist" was a term used to describe the discipline of obtaining and interpreting radiographs. Somewhere along the line, technology advanced, focus groups formed and marketing analysts suggested that this discipline be renamed "imaging." All references to radiologists in Lesson #47 also apply to "imaging" physicians.

The radiologist is not a doctor in the classic sense. He sits in a dark room, living in an abstract world of shadow and innuendo. He is the living medical equivalent of Plato's cave analogy. The radiologist sees reflections of reality, not reality itself. Unlike the radiologist, the surgeon lives in a world of concrete anatomic fact.

"Ordering radiological studies is a medical art ... based on a knowledge of the case, a concern for an anatomic complication and a recognition of what goes on in a radiology department."

Radiologists have the ability to detect disease. Given the exigencies of the X-ray day and the near pandemonium of most X-ray suites, they do not have the time to chase down surgeons or residents prior to doing their studies. This puts them at a disadvantage - a disadvantage easily overcome by providing adequate clinical information to them.

Let us look at some representative X-ray requests recently ordered on a busy surgical service at a major metropolitan hospital with excellent educational facilities and easy freeway access to major recreational areas:

■   Study requested: upper gastrointestinal exam.

Reason given for study: upper abdominal pain. Clinical information *omitted: the patient is six days after a Billroth II reconstruction for a perforated gastric ulcer. The surgical team is concerned about a confined leak or gastric atony.*

■   Study requested: contrast swallow.

Reason given for study: s/p esophagogastrectomy. Clinical information *omitted: the patient is one week after a total gastrectomy for a gastric cancer. An intestinal pouch was created. The team is interested in the status of the anastomosis prior to beginning oral feeding.*

■   Study requested: KUB.

Reason given for study: ?SBO. Clinical information *omitted: the patient underwent an emergency colectomy for a barium enema perforation of the rectum. His ileus persists.*

■   Study requested: sinogram.

Reason given for study: ?fistula. Clinical information *omitted: the patient underwent a low anterior resection with diverting colostomy for a low rectal lesion. The perineum was drained. The drain was removed and feculent material subsequently appeared in the drain site.*

■   Study requested: chest X-ray.

Reason given for study: s/p laparotomy. Clinical information *omitted: the patient underwent an esophagogastrectomy which necessitated opening the left chest for the excision and reconstruction.*

One can easily see from these five examples how the clinical information would have enhanced the quality of the study ordered. Such information provides direction for the radiologist. In the absence of such information, the study (and sometimes the patient) suffers.

Ordering radiological studies is a medical art. It is an art form based on a knowledge of the case, a concern for an anatomic complication and a recognition of what goes on in a radiology department. Developing this art causes the resident or staff surgeon to boil down the problem to a précis of the entire case and to provide direction to the radiologic consultant. Such skillful direction enhances the quality of the studies ordered.

Matrix Lesson 48

There is no law that says that
a colostomy must be closed

Many Matrix discussions are based on complications of colostomy creation or colostomy closure. Colostomies can (and often are) life-saving. Most are temporary. The risks of colostomy closure are generally under-appreciated by surgical residents. He who creates a colostomy is not duty, honor or legally bound to close that colostomy.

The closure of a colostomy has its own set of risks and complications. Recognizing these risks and complications must be figured in to any decision for colostomy closure. Many elderly patients have survived catastrophic illnesses and count each day of survival as a gift. If these patients have undergone colostomy, some are perfectly content to keep that colostomy rather than engender the risk of a second procedure.

A surgeon should not rotely respond to the presence of a stoma with a lock-tight plan for closure. Colostomy closure in the elderly must be put to the patient as an independent procedure with its own set of risks and complications.

Some of these patients will be caught in the "colostomy closure vortex." They are automatically booked for closure at some arbitrary point in the future. Before you can say "Remember Matrix Lesson #48" these patients appear on the operative schedule, suffer a complication and wind up at the Matrix Conference.

The first question is always: did you analyze the risk of colostomy closure in this patient as part of your pre-operative assessment? Despite the relative safety of the procedure, the anesthetic support and the increasing sophistication of surgeons to operate on the elderly, a certain number of patients, after a dispassionate discussion of risk and complication, will defer their closures.

"Colostomy closure in the elderly must be put to the patient as an independent procedure with its own set of risks and complications."

It is just as important to discuss these issues with the referring doctor, some of whom view colostomy closure as a minor procedure without risk or complication.

Oh, I can hear the professors now! "What? This guy is so unsure of his skills that he's letting our senior citizens walk around for life with colostomies!" I refer the professoriate to Matrix Lesson #94 and will let them figure it out for themselves.

A surgeon should use the same thought and risk analysis to a colostomy closure, as he would for any surgical procedure. Assess the patient. Assess the risks and benefits of the procedure. Let the patient and his family have an active role in the decision to reverse or close any colostomy.

Matrix Lesson 49

The modern-day chief of surgery functions as a C.E.O (chief executive officer), not as a C.E.O (chief educational officer)

Current surgical department chiefs bear no resemblance to chiefs of surgery of former days. The chief of a department of surgery today is a C.E.O. - a chief executive officer.

The chief of surgery's *primary* task is to guarantee the financial stability of the department of surgery.

The public thinks of a chief of surgery in the classical sense. They see this kindly Norman Rockwell figure at the bedside, on the ward, rounding with the residents and in the operating theater. The uninitiated see the chief doing those things that one would normally do to participate in the education of young surgeons. They think of him as a healer. Today he is a dealer. The mythical figure of the chief died many years ago.

With the advent of the mega-medical center and the subsequent departmental battles over funding, the education of surgeons has become subordinate to departmental financial goals. With this change, the main job of the chief became departmental management. Primary commitment to and activities in the arena of education were subordinated to divisional administration.

Current chiefs of surgery must make sure that the department is not, as the accountants say, a "cost-loser." That is perhaps the greatest insult that can be hurled at a current chief of surgery. "Yes he can cure cancer. Yes, he has the patience to take an intern through a colectomy. Yes, the residents love him but you know, when you come right down to it - *he's just another cost-loser for the division*." The hospital accountant has just pulled rank on the chief!

"The chief of surgery's primary task is to guarantee the financial stability of the department of surgery."

The need to raise money, conduct research, placate the administration and co-ordinate the ever-burgeoning legions of underlings (see Matrix Lesson #77) leaves no time for the chief of surgery to fulfill traditional surgical educational obligations.

Which is why an understanding of Matrix Lesson #49 is so important. This lesson introduces the reader to the need in every division of surgery for a C.E.O. - a chief educational officer.

Paid like the chief, given a benefits package and a contract like the chief, given space like the chief and given support like the chief, the chief educational officer would do what a classic chief of surgery used to do.

His primary function would be to oversee the surgical education of his division. He would be the object of a search committee who would screen, interview, and assess his *educational skills,* just as the financial and managerial skills of current chiefs are assessed.

Enhanced by his experience and reputation, this chief educational officer would put surgical education on the same level as grants, contracts, and department retreats. There are many surgeons who could fulfill this role. In so doing, these C.E.O.s would revive the spirit of surgical education the current setup is doing its best to push aside.

The resident should never delude himself into thinking that one of the main goals of a current division of surgery is his education. Although the mission statement is tripartite - patient care, research and education - surgical education has been subordinated on the chief's agenda. Fortunately, surgical education is a very personal and individually driven entity which explains why an excellent surgical education can be had in a variety of programs.

Once the resident understands the difference between a chief executive officer and a chief educational officer, he can put his chief's position in perspective and can begin to educate himself.

Perhaps one day current chiefs will master Matrix Lesson #49 and will realize that the literal translation of doctor is .... teacher.

Matrix Lesson 50

If you think about a colostomy,
just *think* about a colostomy

A wizened Boston surgical attending once said to me during a colon resection: "Gordon, if you think about a colostomy during colon surgery, you should *do* a colostomy." This particular attending never spoke.

He never acknowledged the presence of, or, for that matter, the existence of the resident. We were there to serve him and to witness his technical brilliance. The telepathic theory of teaching surgery was very popular in the mid-seventies, particularly among the Harvard crowd.

I do not know why he departed from his customary silence during that particular operation on that particular day. "Gordon, if you think about a colostomy during colon surgery, you should *do* a colostomy" was his single five-year contribution to what is commonly referred to as my "fund of surgical knowledge."

The statement he offered is an old saw handed down from surgical generation to generation. As with most old saws and shopworn surgical statements, it had a germ of truth but is poorly worded and somewhat illogical.

"If you think about a colostomy, you should do a colostomy" never made sense to me. During longer operations, I thought about many things which I would never do. My thoughts usually centered on various members of the nursing staff. Although rather sophomorically stated, I know what that old guy meant. He meant that if there was any doubt in your mind about the integrity of a colon anastomosis, you should divert the colon and should perform a colostomy.

It could have been phrased with much more intelligence and meaning. It could have been so much more insightful and instructive. It could have been laced with experience. But instead, it was reduced to one of those patent professorial edicts that have killed and maimed more people than various international border skirmishes. The statement, by attitude and wording, reduced a salient point of surgical teaching to a cheap slogan.

"... if there was any doubt in your mind about the integrity of a colon anastomosis, you should divert the colon and should perform a colostomy."

If you think about a colostomy, assess the reasons for performing one. If you have a cogent reason, then create a colostomy. Think. Assess. Analyze. Weigh the risks and benefits. Save the knee-jerks for the neurologic examination.

Matrix Lesson 51

New professors of surgery are like newly ordained ministers

I am a student of medical audiences. My favorite is the audience at the Matrix Conference, for reasons which I outlined in the seminal text *Gordon's Guide to the Surgical Morbidity and Mortality Conference* (Philadelphia: Hanley & Belfus, 1994).

I study the audience reactions and comments, as well as their interactions with other audience members. Of all of the members of the typical medical audience, none is more fascinating to study than the genus *professorius neophytus surgiensis* (the young professor of surgery).

Perhaps he has just finished a fellowship. Perhaps he has made his mark in the lab and is now new to the current group. Perhaps he is the "fair-haired" boy, the king-designate of the department. Perhaps she is the rising star in the local surgical firmament. Maybe he has come from another institution, a fact which assures that every statement which comes out of his mouth for the next five years will begin: "At (former institution), we always did it this way ..." Maybe he just married the chief's daughter. Maybe he just married the chief! Maybe he is a surgical program rain-maker with the potential for making huge profits for the department.

"The defining characteristic of this surgical arriviste is the assumption of instant credibility because of the mantle of the professoriate."

There is no more enjoyable activity than to study him as he feels his way through the current surgical terrain. These observations become even more interesting if the new arrival is a graduate of the program in which he now serves as an attending surgeon.

The defining characteristic of this surgical arriviste is the assumption of instant credibility because of the mantle of the professoriate.

The definitive study of the surgical professoriate and its role in surgery today is currently being written.* In this text there is a chapter on new professors. This chapter discusses in detail the aura surrounding them. This text discusses professorial demeanor, keys to career advancement and the interplay between the young professor and the rank and file of his division. This text will be the definitive resource for future surgical archaeologists.

Many analogies can be made to professions in which the title itself gives instant credibility to the holder of that title. No comparison is more

* Gordon's Guide to the Surgical Professoriate.

fitting than comparing the new professor of surgery to a newly ordained minister.

Mencken said it best: "... the young divine is a safe and distinguished man the moment he is ordained; indeed, his popularity especially among the faithful who are fair, is often greater at that moment than it ever is afterward. His livelihood is assured instantly. At one stroke, he becomes a person of dignity and importance, eminent in his community, deferred to even by those who question his magic, and vaguely and pleasantly feared by those who credit it." **

If one substitutes "young professor" for "divine" in Mencken's description, one will have the essence of this position in the department of surgery.

Matrix Lesson #51 is a guide for placing new professors into perspective. Knowledge of this lesson saves time and energy as one negotiates the political byways of the medical center.

** Mencken HL. *The American Mercury*. June 1924: 183. From *A Mencken Chrestomathy*. His Own Selection of his Choicest Writings. Vintage Books edition, 1982: 73-5.

Matrix Lesson 52

Get the old records

Perhaps this lesson should just be a corollary of Lesson #8 which states that last year's study, reportedly normal, is always abnormal. But Matrix Lesson #52 is wider in its application and certainly in its spirit.

The spirit of Matrix Lesson #52 is the spirit of intellectual curiosity coupled with the underpinning of surgery - attention to detail and verification of fact. One of the most frequent questions posed to a presenting resident at the Matrix Conference is: "Did you review the old records?"

The world has caught up to the surgical "day". We now have twenty-four-hour copy services, electronic mail, the World Wide Web and even ESPN2.

"The old records are your greatest ally in solving problems in patients who have had previous surgery or hospitalizations."

It is now possible to retrieve old records at any time and under any circumstances. The world of information never sleeps. Getting old records relies on the four "Fs" of surgical record retrieval. *

■   Fone.

Here we are at the millennium, able to place two men into orbit to fix a mirror. Why, then, cannot a resident pick up a telephone (charging the cost of the call to the department) and call a record room in another city for operative records?

Why, then, cannot an interested resident call a surgeon in another city and say: "Dr. Smith, we have your patient here in the ER. Could you tell us what operation you performed on him a few years ago?"

The telephone is a great ally in record retrieval of data for patients who cannot give a history, whose history is suspect, or whose previous surgeries are unknown.

■   Fax.

Not only can we get low-level medical record types to read to us over the phone, but we can actually obtain these documents by the fax machine.

---

* Adapted from Gordon LA. *Gordon's Guide to the Surgical Morbidity and Mortality Conference.* Philadelphia: Hanley & Belfus, 1994. Reproduced with permission from Elsevier.

It may come as a shock that the fax machine can actually be used for efforts other than football pools! Operative reports, clinic visits, pathology reports, or X-ray reports can all be faxed to the appropriate place.

Every house-staff lounge, department headquarters, surgical lounge or resident office has a fax machine. Even the dreaded HIPPA mandated "release of record" form can be faxed to the record rooms around the world.

There is not a medical records person alive who can withstand the onslaught of: "Look this is a medical emergency. Please fax that operative report now or I'll have to page your supervisor." This works every time, even though it is not really an emergency and the responsible resident just wants to look good at the Matrix Conference.

People are amazed that the appendectomy was never done, that there was some real question whether or not Crohn's disease was present, or in fact that there were no findings of a bowel obstruction at the surgery for a bowel obstruction. These are significant points, all of which are retrievable with a little spirit, enthusiasm and tenacity.

■ Fellowship.

This word was in vogue in the halcyon days of American surgery. There was a time when the discipline of surgery was a calling rather than a trade.

Fellowship was a feeling of camaraderie among surgeons that led to *esprit de corps*, a sense of mutual respect and most important, a sense of brotherly (or sisterly) helpfulness.

If one were to call a surgeon in another city, that spirit of fellowship would mean that that doctor would take the time to recollect the case, share the problems encountered in performing or diagnosing the problem, and would actually help the caller. He would shed new light on the complication with which the new team was wrestling. He might even fax or send the records himself. Surgical fellowship can be an important part of record retrieval.

▪   Fed-Ex™.

I am not a Fedex share-holder. No-one in my family or circle of friends has any relationship to the company. I can now state, within the bounds of current "conflict of interest" laws and with a clear conscience, that Fedex has probably contributed more to the care of surgical patients than many grants.

Was it cancer? Was it Crohn's? The presenting resident would be wise to call and get the slides from the Pathology Department of the original facility. Call and get the entire record if there is too much to fax.

How about X-rays? They can be shipped overnight. Why the "Collected Hits of Richard Clayderman" arrives next-day air, and yet the critical CAT scan of a moribund patient languishes in a basement gathering dust is the kind of surgical dilemma the professoriate should be working on!

The Four Fs are the basis for Matrix Lesson #52. The old records are your greatest ally in solving problems in patients who have had previous surgery or hospitalizations.

Matrix Lesson 53

The "senior" author had nothing to do with the article to which his name is affixed

---

"The multiauthored article is the standard in the medical sciences, where the politics of the laboratory and the academy often loom larger than the singularity of the argument or grace of its execution." *

* Suzanne Poirer, PhD. Charting the Chart - An Exercise in Interpretation(s). *Literature and Medicine* 1992; 11(1): 1.

Presentations at the Matrix Conference often include references to the surgical literature. When the resident puts up his reference slide, the title and data are usually dwarfed by a half-page list of authors. The knowledgeable reader often wonders: "Who is the 'senior author' of this paper?"

There are many similarities between the "senior author" and the "senior surgeon" (see Matrix Lesson #93). Both are amorphous concepts magically bestowed on surgeons. Neither has rigorous qualifiers. These are titles that enhance the people they describe. These titles convey experience, involvement and sagacity.

But there is a major difference between the two. "Senior surgeon" is merely a name and a concept which is at least, even if only in the mind of the surgeon, intellectually honest. The surgeon really believes that he is a senior surgeon. He has performed surgery in the past and may be performing surgery now. At the least, he is participating in the endeavor of surgery.

Not so with many of the "senior" authors. In many cases, the title "senior author" is a bona fide fraud. The senior author of many papers in the literature has his name on the paper out of courtesy, fear, or, in a very few cases, respect for past performance. He usually has little to do with the actual writing of the paper, other than saying in the resident's lounge: "Wouldn't it be nice if someone wrote a paper on ...."

The major impact of the concept of the senior author is environmental, not medical. The amount of paper used for these publications is destroying untold numbers of trees. I am surprised that some environmentally conscious surgical resident has not exposed this by now, but I suppose there are job security issues. Surgical authorship is out of control!

Three surgeons can't sit down for coffee without walking away with plans for a new journal. Since the engine of academia and pseudo-academia (the academia of my life) is publishing, the philosophy is that if an already existing journal with its own network of acceptance exists, why beat one's head against a wall? Get your own journal and publish your own papers! Or, more importantly, the papers of your friends.

A recent review of the "List of Referenced Journals" volume of the Index Medicus runs about two hundred pages. There are, on average, thirty journals listed on each page. That totals approximately six thousand journals. Most of these are monthly publications.

Now physicians are a pretty smart group. But is there enough original thought likely to benefit humanity to justify 4,800 medical journals? Here are some journal titles of interest. (If I may use a Dave Barry term) - I am not kidding!

- *Andrologica.*
  (I thought this was a Greco-Roman folk poem like Beowulf!)
- *Archives of Environmental Contamination.*
  (Written by the housekeeper in charge of the residents' lounge.)
- *Annals of Physiological Anthropology.*
  (Studying the bodily function of dead people. This is unlikely to benefit anyone currently in my Department, although I have some concerns about a few members.)
- *American Journal of Ortho-Psychiatry.*
  (Catering to mentally disturbed orthopedic surgeons.)
- *Australasian Physical and Engineering Sciences in Medicine.*
  (Edited by Paul Hogan.)

These multiple journals are the units of senior authorship. They are the chits on the game-board of medical-academic advancement. They serve one purpose only - to exponentially fatten the curriculum vitae (see Matrix Lesson #85). To fully appreciate the principles behind Matrix Lesson #53, we must define some terms:

- Authorship - n., state of an individual with faint familiarity with a scientific paper bearing his name.
- First author - n., outlined the paper, usually on the back of a progress note sheet.
- Second author - n., paid for the Xeroxing of the references.
- Third author - n, walked through the room where the paper was being written.

- Fourth author - n., has office in same building where paper was written.
- Fifth author - n., writes recommendations for authors 1-4.
- Senior author - n., has a loose, although senior position to authors 1-5 and is responsible for their career advancement.
- Acknowledged individual - responsible for writing the paper.

As a practical exercise in interpreting lesson #53 let's dissect a typical reference, in an attempt to further define the role of the senior author:

Gordon LA, Auerbach A (Red), Lombardi VA, Belichick W, and Jones KC. Anatomic Correlates in Pancreatic Surgery - Syntax, Simile and Synechiae. *Am J Anat Acta Physiolog Rheumatologica Scandinavica* (Dansk outlet) Supple. 2003; II: 148-54.

- Gordon LA - the "first author" - the grunt, the slave, the scrivener, the only one:
  a) who really worked on the paper;
  b) who knows the contents of the paper; and
  c) who has read the paper.
- Auerbach A (Red) - the attending who suggested the paper.
- Lombardi VA - the surgeon who was assisting on the case when it was suggested that the paper be written.
- Belichick W - the surgeon whose secretary typed the paper.
- Jones KC - the Department Chairman, or person with the most influence over the second author, i.e. the senior author.

It is extremely easy, particularly for residents, to test the validity of lesson #53. Try this. Retrieve a paper from the institution in which the resident is enrolled. Get the senior author's name. Go up to him and say: "Professor Nodlinger, I enjoyed your recent paper in the *Journal of Inane Ramblings*, but one thing bothered me. How did you reconcile the data in Table III with the photograph?"

The blank look generated by this question is a testament to the value of Matrix Lesson #53.

Matrix Lesson 54

Never refer to an operation as "just a ....."

I learned this particular lesson in 1978 when, during rounds, I asked the intern what had happened the night before. His reply was prophetic: "Just an appy."

"Just an appy" left the hospital three months later after four operations and a cardiac arrest. "Just an appy" occupied the protocol for several Matrix Conferences. "Just an appy" was the main topic of discussion on the surgical service for about a year. Overall, "just an appy" was an unhappy experience for all involved.

Each operation in surgery has its own set of risks and potential complications. Thankfully, most of the time, due to the skill of the surgeon and the overwhelming power of the fibroblast, things go well. People heal, recover and go about their lives.

But every operation, from the excision of a sebcaeous cyst under local anesthesia as an outpatient, to a pancreatic head resection, has the potential for life-threatening and morbid complication.

Every operation!

It is important to respect this potential for death and misery inherent in each of our operations. Knowledge of the procedure and all of its postoperative complications leads to that respect.

"Any procedure in surgery can result in a horrible complication. The vagaries of human biology assure this."

Herein lies the charge to surgical educators and attending surgeons. The intern who called it "just an appy" to some degree was reflecting his own limited experience. He had never seen a pelvic abscess. He had never cared for a patient in septic shock. The concepts of cecal fistulization, septic pelvic thrombophlebitis, wound dehiscence, gastro-intestinal stress bleed, necrotizing fasciitis, postoperative small bowel obstruction and subclavian vein thrombosis, were familiar to him, but out of the realm of his comprehension when linked to an appendectomy. These entities were, for him, theory. They became frighteningly real.

Using the phrase "Just an ..." reflects a lack of appreciation for surgical pathology. Any procedure in surgery can result in a horrible complication. The vagaries of human biology assure this.

Surgical procedures are not chemistry experiments with a uniformly predictable outcome. Each procedure must be approached with a respect for the multiple responses human physiology may have to any insult.

If Lesson #54 is not observed on your service, the appropriate penalty is to have the offender go to the medical library. He or she is then responsible for the appropriate chapter in Hardy: *Complications in Surgery and Their Management* (Philadelphia: Saunders, 1981). This magnificent (though somewhat dated) compilation of the potential ills of every procedure we do should be part of every intern packet distributed in July. By the end of the academic year, this classic text will have been mastered by several members of the surgical team.

I assure you that they will never refer to any operation as "just a ..." They will have learned Matrix Lesson #54.

Matrix Lesson 55

Never ask this question: "What kind of incision should we make?"

Before there was reason and intelligence in clinical surgery and certainly well before the laparoscopic revolution, there was the debate about the type of incision to be used.

In some quarters, this debate still rages. I remember standing at the operating table, across from one of my chief residents. He began: "Gordon, what type of incision should we use here? The paramedian, the transverse, the chevron, the midline, the muscle-splitting, the muscle retracting, the McBurney, the Rocky-Davis or the Stewart?" I felt as if I were in a restaurant and had to choose from the list of specials.

Many surgical incisions are named after the famous people who designed and used them. And I use the word "design" advisedly, since making an incision consists of placing the knife on the abdomen, dragging it and pushing it into the flesh. This is not a particularly challenging task, and does not take an inordinate amount of surgical skill to master.

There is one defining characteristic of surgeons who belabor discussions regarding incision placement - *none of them know really what to do once the incision has been made!*

These surgeons have specialized, as it were, in incision placement. That is their forte. They have expended so much time and mental effort into reasoning through an "incision decision" that that effort has become a stand-alone entity. Once the incision has been chosen, these surgeons have no intellectual reserve left to deal with the real issues of the surgery at hand.

"The midline is embryologically and surgically logical. Its perfect evolutionary history begs surgeons to use it."

Ideally, after debating, analyzing and deciding on which of the myriad of surgical incisions to make, these surgeons should leave the operating theater. They should let another surgeon perform the operation.

The great debate over incisions began in the early years of laparotomy. In typical surgical fashion, after describing a particular incision, the surgeon did not give it an easily recognizeable anatomic name. The surgeon gave it *his* name.

This ploy was an early effort at surgical marketing. Doctor Wilson now had to admit, and even dictate in his own operative report that he used the incision of his two greatest competitors, Rocky and Davis.

Competitors of Dr. Weir now had to use his name as they extended their appendectomy incisions. It was the first example of medical self-promotion.

"Yes, I'm Professor Parker and he's Professor Kehr!* Let's see, why not make the incision here and, oh, yes, we'll call it - let me see. Let's give it an anatomically precise name that will let everyone know the reason for making it. Let me see, oh, I've got it! We'll call it the Parker-Kehr incision!"

On and on, year after year, surgeon after surgeon - Kocher, Cheatle-Henry, Rocky-Davis, Rocky III, Al Davis, Bialystok-Bloom, - on and on, naming incisions and creating a confusing collection of names where no confusion need exist.

Which brings me to the embryology of the human midline. The amazing evolution of the intra-abdominal contents ended with a gift wrap sealed at the midline. The blastomeres, somatosomes, anlagen (ventral and dorsal) and primitive tubes had all completed their evolutionary tasks. What would top it off? A Rocky-Davis? A paramedian? No! What topped it off as the crowning evolutionary glory of visceral humankind was: the midline. The midline is embryologically and surgically logical. Its perfect evolutionary history begs surgeons to use it.

I am introducing a bill into the State Legislature (House Bill #M-9865 - Felonious Use of Non-Midline Incisions) that makes anything other than a midline incision illegal. Once passed, this should settle the issue and eliminate forever the annoying question that, by following Matrix Lesson #55, should never be asked.

* Try singing this as if in a Gilbert and Sullivan musical.

Matrix Lesson 56

Never use subjective terms in a medical history

Residents have learned some bad linguistic habits over the years in keeping with the general decline of English usage. They will often weave these bad habits into their Matrix presentations. They forget that the surgical history and physical should look as if it were written by Dr. Jack Webb* - just the facts.

Unfortunately (vide infra), several subjective terms have become ingrained in the medical historical jargon. If one examines their meanings one will cease using them and thus will add to the specificity and overall value of medical histories and formal presentations.

---

* The style of Jack Webb is seen nightly on cable television as *Dragnet* is rebroadcast. It should be required viewing for all medical residents.

Let's look at these examples, culled from recent Matrix presentations:

▓   This thirty-five-year-old Caucasian *gentleman* .....

Gentleman: a man who demonstrates his gentle (noble) birth by appropriate behavior or moral qualities: chivalrous conduct, consideration for others, sense of honor.

I know some fairly perceptive physicians who use this term, yet I doubt if they realize what they imply by the term "gentleman." It never made sense to me to use this term after knowing someone for 20-30 minutes, particularly when that someone may be a perpetrator sleeping under a freeway overpass (or over a freeway underpass).

While gentlemen may inhabit such areas, it is unlikely that they have maintained the characteristics of a noble birth. The term "gentleman" is, as the definition shows, quite specific. It describes more than can be learned from an interview for medical reasons.

▓   This *lovely* 20-year-old female Filipino nursing student ....

Lovely: loving, kind, affectionate; worthy of love; suited to attract love; spiritually or morally beautiful; exquisitely beautiful.

"Using the[se] subjective terms ... turns a scientific document (the medical history) into a collection of unscientific semantically inappropriate adjectives."

The term "gentleman" makes me apoplectic. An even more egregious departure from sane medical descriptive terminology is the term "lovely." This term induces oculo-gyric crises.

How can this term ever be used in a medical history? Here we are in the middle of an analysis of right lower quadrant pain, and the responsible physician becomes Alfred Lord Tennyson. He waxes poetic on the nuances of female beauty. How can one describe the spiritual or moral beauty of a young woman in pain? Is this medicine or metaphysics?

■   This *unfortunate* 83-year-old African-American male ....

Unfortunate: not favored by fortune; suffering misfortune, unlucky, unhappy; an unfortunate person, specifically a woman engaged in prostitution.

Medicine, particularly surgery, has as its charge the alleviation of human suffering. We deal with the touchstone of suffering - pain. We have no insight into fortune, fate or luck. We are thrust into situations and must assess them in terms of their science, not their position in the cosmos. Using the term *unfortunate* means we substitute palmistry for dispassionate scientific thought.

We now come to the touchstone word - the word which most clearly reveals ignorance of Matrix Lesson #56. The word, which when seen sends semantic shivers throughout my body. The word which I search for, as if it were the holy grail of illogical medical description. The word which, when written by a surgical resident, assures him of many trips to the bowels of the medical library to present to me on rounds a brief biographical vignette of Gregor, Friedrich Trendelenberg's liveryman! That word .... that word .... that word: delightful.

■   This *delightful* 76-year-old Caucasian female was in her usual state of .....

Delightful: the fact or condition of being delighted; pleasure, joy or gratification felt in a high degree. A thing which, or person, who causes great pleasure or joy.

All definitions of delightful dwell on the high degree of pleasure, joy or rapture induced by the object being described. If something is delightful, it is not just pleasurable; it is *highly* pleasurable to the point of rapture or ecstasy. To be delightful is to be, in fact, beyond the bounds of what is normally pleasurable.

I enjoy my work. I derive a great deal of professional satisfaction from it. Yet, I have never been confronted with a clinical history, past medical history, review of systems or a physical examination that led me to conclude that the patient was delightful.

Call me old-fashioned, but I never entered a state of rapture after interviewing a new patient. Let's talk delightful. Pamela Anderson, as a stand alone conceptual entity, is delightful. Mozart's bassoon concerto in B flat is delightful. Beethoven's sonata #25 in G is delightful. Vivaldi's flute concerto in G minor is delightful (a patient gave me classical CDs last Christmas). Doubling down on an ace-eight when the dealer is showing a five with a plus count and being dealt a two as the casino goes crazy is delightful. A tax credit is delightful. These are rapturous occasions. But a 76-year-old female sporting a salem sump tube? I don't think so!

Using the subjective terms listed above turns a scientific document (the medical history) into a collection of unscientific, semantically inappropriate adjectives. These words should not be used.

Matrix Lesson #56 teaches us that these words should not be used in the medical record.

Note: definitions are from *The New Shorter Oxford English Dictionary*. Oxford: Clarendon Press, 1993.

Matrix
Lesson 57

A surgeons' lounge should reflect the
demeanor of the surgeons who use it

The first surgeons' lounge I entered was in a Chicago teaching hospital. That lounge had been built in the later years of the nineteenth century. The room was dimly lit. The walls were paneled with dark weathered wood. Bookcases full of classic surgical texts lined the walls. The chairs were comfortable leather-cushioned affairs. Ikea was but a dream. The light fixtures were bronze with dark green glass covering the bulbs. The room was carpeted. Classical music played softly from a radio in the corner. Framed portraits of former chiefs of surgery with their years of service engraved beneath their names hung on the wall. Chicago dailies were on a low table in the center of the room. A silver coffee service was in the corner. There was the faint smell of cigars. The room took on a powerful aura, particularly in the early morning of a Chicago winter. The essence of surgery emanated from that surgeons' lounge. The room was stately, serious and steeped in history.

I knew then that I wanted to become a surgeon. I knew upon entering that room that I would try to use that room's atmosphere to set the tone for my own professional work.

The room that readies a surgeon for his daily work should be carefully designed and planned. The room should reflect the surgeon's commitment to his craft and should set the tone for how that commitment is realized.

Sadly, most surgeons' lounges are not designed by surgeons. They seem to be designed by failed architects whose last project was the East Moline Correctional Facility.

"However, the surgeons' lounge is a special place, setting the tone for a special task."

I am as aware as the next surgeon of budgetary restrictions and the rampant departmental egalitarianism coursing through medical centers today. However, the surgeons' lounge is a special place, setting the tone for a special task. An appreciation of this should lead to better designed surgeons' lounges.

Redesigning your surgeons' lounge is rather easy. It can be done inexpensively. I work at a large hospital which was designed (I think) by an architect. That architect knew nothing about surgeons' lounges, so he simply built a locker room. The room has the characteristics of a holding tank, usually seen in the final minutes of "America's Most Wanted." The room is a cold, lifeless, fluorescently-lit, white-tiled affair, conducive to intramural basketball, but certainly not to surgery.

Several years ago, I took on as my mission a redesign of that lounge. My attempt through formal hospital channels failed shortly after I was presented with requisition #56-P9843 - Inter-Departmental Request. This document had to go through committee and had to be signed by three members of the administration and the Chief of the Department of Surgery.

It was clear to me that I had to get more practical. I called a former patient who worked in "Plant Engineering." I called a friend who worked in the audiovisual department. I called a person who owed me something, who happened to work in the electrical department. And finally, I called Sol. Sol is the person you go to get something done, but it costs you. Thankfully, for every large institution, there is always a Sol.

I solicited a few donations from my colleagues and within three weeks we had: carpeting, classical music, framed greats of clinical surgery, and even a television with a remote control next to a couch. With four phone calls, a modest cash outlay and an appreciation of the importance of the surgeons' lounge, the task was completed. The surgeons in my division now prepare for their day's work in a proper place conducive to study and reflection. Instead of feeling that they are facing arraignment, they feel enthused, uplifted and confident that their day's activities will be performed in the grand tradition of clinical surgery.

The needed coffee-maker and the daily papers are being discussed by representatives of a prominent medical device company, but I am having trouble assuring them that our Division will order seven beam coagulators.

Matrix Lesson 58

Use as much surgical Yiddish as possible

Yiddish words could frequently be heard in early Matrix Conferences, particularly the plaintive "oy vey!" as the resident related some illogical act.

Matrix Lesson #58 is a plea to maintain Yiddish in certain surgical situations. Yiddish is tailor-made to express many emotions which may arise in those situations. Although anatomic nomenclature is quite specific, universally recognized and a basic part of surgery, our surgical language is somewhat limited in specific circumstances. Yiddish helps in those surgical circumstances which require special emphasis.

Yiddish is a combination of several languages. Many Yiddish words have found their way into the English language. Surgery is a very emotional discipline and Yiddish is a very emotional language. To a large semantic degree, they were made for each other.

I am in the process of writing the definitive (is there any other kind?) book, *Yiddish for Surgeons*. This text will make the following words common on the surgical services of the world, even on those services with affiliations not used to such words.

▦   Bopkis - n., of no value; nothing; of no significance.

Example #1: "We explored her for appendicitis, but found *bopkis*."

Example #2: "The red-cell scan means *bopkis* in this case."

Bopkis refers to an insignificant finding, or to an absence of surgical pathology. The term is also used to describe what divorced surgeons are left with after their settlements. The most enjoyable usage of this word is when it is used to tell children what is left to them in wills.

▦   Tsuris - n., trouble

Example: While exploring a patient for a pancreatic mass, the operating surgeon discovers that the tumor is infiltrating the transverse mesocolon and the superior mesenteric artery. He looks at the surgical team and states: "This patient has real *tsuris*!"

All medicine is divided into two parts: tsuris major and tsuris minor. Tsuris minor refers to such entities as an infiltrated intravenous line, a superficial phlebitis or a viral gastroenteritis. Tsuris major, on the other hand, refers to unresectable tumors, exsanguinating gastrointestinal hemorrhage or to a toxic megacolon. A famous reference work describing this classification is Roget's "Tsuris."

▦   Zaftig - adj., hefty, thick, stout.

Example: "The patient was not obese. She was *zaftig*."

This word describes the nether region between hefty and obese. It does not carry the negative connotation of obese. It has a certain healthy and desirable characteristic. If you ever see a "Z" on the label of a dress in a store for larger women, you now know what it means.

▧   Megillah - n., a long and involved story.

Example #1: "What is this - a case presentation or a *megillah*?"

Example #2: "Give me the essential points of the case. I don't want the whole *megillah*!"

Internists live for the megillah. In their eyes a megillah is an intellectual exercise of great value to the patient and the consulting doctor.

Surgeons see the megillah for what it really is - a lofty verbal exaltation of a few essential facts designed to impress the listener with length rather than with substance. This word has special meaning for the resident presenting at the Matrix Conference. We live in an age of short attention span. Present the essential facts and findings of the case. Get to the point!

"Yiddish helps in those surgical circumstances which require special emphasis."

▧   Mazel tov! - expletive, Good luck!

Example: Surgeon #1: "My Whipple resection sailed! Home in eight days!"

Surgeon #2: "*Mazel tov!*"

Mazel tov is another common Yiddish surgical expletive used to confer good luck in specific situations. Births, bar mitzvahs, the achievement of board certification, defense verdicts or unusual cases that go well are often responded to by a colleague with a hearty mazel tov!

A linguistic nuance becoming more common is to use this expletive to stare danger, death and destruction squarely in the face. In this instance it is used to wish good luck when good luck is sorely needed.

Examples:
Surgeon #1: "My wife is sleeping with my partner."
"My partner stole from me."
"They revoked my privileges."
"The anterior resection I did last Thursday is leaking."

Surgeon #2: "*Mazel tov!*"

■ Tsimmis n., a complicated or burdensome situation; a big deal; a major production.

Example #1: "Branson did a hernia yesterday. He makes a *tsimmis* out of every case!"

Example #2: Surgeon #1: "What took you so long?"

Surgeon #2: "The case began as an appendectomy, but it turned into a big *tsimmis*."

A tsimmis arises in two specific medical situations. The most common situation occurs when the surgeon is confronted with unusual, unexpected or difficult surgical findings. For example: a confined ruptured appendix with dense adhesions; an inflammatory aneurysm; a cholecystectomy with unexpected bile duct stones; or a colectomy with tumor adherence to the ureter. In these situations, a relatively straightforward case becomes more complicated. These situations widen the scope of the procedure and in so doing increase its complexity. The case becomes a tsimmis.

A tsimmis can also form through the creative description of a straightforward case. Some surgeons feel the need to increase the complexity of their cases verbally even if they are straightforward anatomically. What they describe postoperatively may bear little resemblance to what they found intra-operatively. There are deep-seated Freudian reasons for this - reasons best left for the psycho-analysts to explain. For example, a relatively routine repair of a sliding indirect inguinal hernia may evolve into a lengthy description of the "intimacy of the colonic serosa with the posterior wall of the sac." Or the repair - basically closing a hole - may be described to colleagues as the Czezlaw-Magruder modification of a Cheatle Henry type IV imbricating interposition Smeadly-Jones pants-over-vest far-near-near-far transition repair. In other words, the surgeon creates a tsimmis out of the hernia repair.

One will also hear the term "big tsimmis" - a favorite term of my father who first used it after my mother asked him to explain the facts of life to me. I remember him saying, "I don't want to make a big tsimmis out of this, but I want to talk to you about something ..."

This is redundant. If you have made a tsimmis out of something, it is already big. I mention big tsimmis only to condemn its use, particularly at grand rounds or national meetings. Using Yiddish terms in the hospital livens up a presentation.

At the risk of creating a megillah, I will end this discussion of Matrix Lesson #58.

Matrix Lesson 59

The progress notes are for the patient's problems, not for the doctor's problems

Matrix presentations always involve a review of the patient's full hospital record. The presenting resident had to review the chart, glean the salient facts and prepare the presentation. The progress notes form a central part of that review. Matrix Lesson #59 concerns itself with the content of those progress notes.

The progress notes are for the recordation of the patient's progress. They are meant to reflect the thinking of the physician or consultant caring for the patient. (By the way there is an ongoing Talmudic debate: should a doctor write a progress note if no progress has been made?)

It seems that many physicians and residents think that the progress notes are sort of note-pads for the documentation of the evolving medical mind. Travel down any corridor on medical teaching services and one will see row upon row of earnest types writing in the charts.

The patients are sleeping. The hospital has wound down. What are these young doctors writing? They are the twenty-first century equivalent of the monks in the scriptorium. Only they are not creating gilt-printed bibles. They are, for the most part, scribbling non-sequitors in a legal document. This makes no sense.

> "Tightly written, specific progress notes with clearly laid out plans and likely causes of problems aid the progress of the patient."

The resident's problem is that he is trying to learn medicine. That is not the patient's problem. The resident's cognitive* problems should not appear in the progress notes. They are progress notes, not works in progress!

Let's examine two examples from a recently reviewed chart:

- Bp 130/80 P=84 R=12
  Squinting in right eye
  ?pupil dilated
  Feels better? Psychological overlay? Could this be conversion reaction?
  Abd. firm, patient hungry
  Plan: MRI

This note reminds me of Wheel of Fortune where you have to guess the phrase or word from disparate letters. Instead of letters, here we

* I use this word without the permission of the American Board of Internal Medicine.

have random thoughts poorly expressed. This resident has more problems than the patient.

▦   Rising WBC
     Falling Hct
     Na+ = 135
     Plan: see orders

This is real progress! The white count is rising. The hematocrit is falling and the sodium is normal. This particular note reminds me of the Rosetta stone. What does it mean? Who can unlock its mystery?

The progress note is not the place for editorializing, confabulating or pontificating. It is not the place for third year students visiting from New York to demonstrate for all mankind that they can list 23 causes of right upper quadrant pain.

In addition to being a much reviewed legal document, the progress notes are meant to review and assess, as well as to relay important information about the patient. Tightly written, specific progress notes with clearly laid out plans and likely causes of problems aid the progress of the patient. Poorly written, wordy free-association word salads confuse the reader and obfuscate the problems of the patient. If Matrix Lesson #59 is learned, the size of the medical record will shrink while its value will increase.

Matrix
Lesson 60

Master the techniques for local anesthesia

"Wha d'ya mean 'master the
technique of local anesthesia'?
Ya just draw up some local and stick it in.
Use a lot and that's that! What's the problem?"

Such is the abysmal state of teaching local anesthesia.
I am a notorious operating theater lizard. I slither from
room to room observing my colleagues, announcing
surprise visits from the medical board. I observe the give-
and-take between resident and attending. Because of
this habit, I have become a frequent witness to the
"drape wave" - that mysterious undulating drape
phenomenon that appears during the early part of cases
performed under local anesthesia.

The drape wave is a combination move created by a shifting patient and a scrambling anesthesiologist. It results in a scenario mimicking an operation on a storm-tossed aircraft carrier during heavy shelling.

"The effective and skillful use of local anesthesia is a surgical art that must be mastered if the surgeon is to use it effectively."

The drape wave often arises from a lack of appreciation for the technique of administration of local anesthesia. Many of our surgical procedures are now done under local anesthesia, yet many surgeons remain unschooled in the art and science of its administration.

The effective and skillful use of local anesthesia is a surgical art that must be mastered if the surgeon is to use it effectively. I was taught by a master - my dentist. Most surgeons regard local anesthesia as the random injection of local anesthetic in an operative area. This is wrong. It is an affront to the American Board of Local Anesthesia (ABLA) and is a disservice to the patients.

There are several elements to the mastery of local anesthesia administration:

■ Realize that the patient is awake.

The surgeon must realize that the patient under local is, usually, awake. The surgeon's voice inflection, demeanor and conduct are different than if the patient were asleep. The surgeon should stay in contact with the patient, telling the patient what he is doing.

It is most reassuring (I know this from a patient's point of view) to have a surgeon who explains what he is doing in non-technical terms. The fact that the patient is being addressed makes him feel at ease.

▓   The size of the needle is important, especially for the initial injection.

The smallest needle hurts the least. (I believe it was Torquemada who first stated this principle of operative surgery.) Injection using a 27-gauge needle is barely perceptible.

▓   The initial speed of injection of the anesthetic is important.

The slower the better. (I believe it was Dr. Ruth who first expounded this principle.)

▓   The surgeon's approach to the tissue and other structures are different under local anesthesia than the approach under a general anesthetic.

The surgeon must have "tissue sense" (see Matrix Lesson #82): the ability to know what he can do to what tissue under a variety of circumstances.

Cleaning off and identifying the pubic tubercle during a hernia repair under local anesthesia is very different from the same maneuver done under general anesthesia. All the men in the recovery room with ice-packs between their legs know this.

▓   Not everyone is a candidate for local anesthesia.

This is a pre-operative judgment which, if wrong, makes for a frustrated surgeon, an unhappy patient and an anesthesiologist who must be readily familiar with the surgical principle of *geschlafen*.*

In every surgical program there are one or two surgeons who have mastered the techniques of local anesthesia. It is obvious to the surgical residents who they are. Residents will contribute immeasurably to their surgical education if they spend some time with these surgeons. These residents will learn firsthand the foundation for Matrix Lesson #60.

---

*Yiddish word meaning "go to sleep."

Matrix Lesson 61

Never ask this question: "Should you remove the appendix?"

Some surgeons attending the weekly Matrix Conference feel compelled to ask questions. They feel obligated to speak. When the scientific analysis is over and when the discussion of surgical principles has ended, these participants are left with only one question: "Should you have removed the appendix?"

In the pantheon of inane surgical questions, "Should we remove the appendix?" holds a hallowed place. It is the first bona fide surgical annoyance with which most surgical residents will be confronted. This question will usually be asked during a case which has nothing to do with the appendix.

In all probability, it will be the first operating room question a resident will be asked while scrubbing on a case. This question is usually asked by the least respected attending surgeon, groping for academic respectability on his service.

Why these surgeons ask this particular question is a source of endless fascination for me. As I come to the conclusion of my long study of this question, I realize that there are a number of my colleagues who feel that their intellectual and surgical stature is enhanced by asking the unanswerable, by pondering the imponderable and by opining on the unopineable. This particular question is the gold standard for the unanswerable arcana of surgery.

I would suggest to the reader to master the answerable before the unanswerable. It is much more practical.

"[this] appendiceal question is inane, illegitimate and unnecessary.
It represents surgical arcana and all of the elements of professorial tautology."

Knowing the length of the human colon is important. That number is a scientific fact likely to help someone some day. The number of grams of fat per cubic centimeter in the lipid solution is a number - a concrete irrefutable fact. Surgical approaches to the indeterminate pancreatic head mass require solid surgical knowledge based on fact and accepted techniques. These answers and their questions rely on a definable fund of knowledge.

Let us examine the thought process of the average surgical resident confronted with this question: "Should we remove the appendix?"

"Let's see. If I say 'yes', the attending will browbeat me about incidental procedures, the risk of infection weighed against the risk of developing appendicitis, and the myriad complications which may follow appendectomy. I better not answer 'yes'. But wait ...

"If I say 'no', he will then ask me the natural history of incidental carcinoids and the likelihood of developing appendicitis in the future. Then he will embark on a tirade on how easy it is and the putative benefits of doing it. He will then crush me and make me a moist spot on the operating room floor by impugning my surgical maturity and inferring that I am afraid of widening the scope of my procedure for the benefit of the patient. He will think me surgically timid. I better not answer 'no'."

How to answer? How to answer? The appendiceal question is inane, illegitimate and unnecessary. It represents surgical arcana and all of the elements of professorial tautology. The appendiceal question belongs in a freshman philosophy class, not in our operating theaters. This question is the stuff of professorships, not the stuff of working surgeons.

I would suggest the following approach should you ever be present when this question is asked.

Attending surgeon to resident half-way through a sigmoid resection: "Well, Dr. Chen, should we remove the appendix?"

Dr. Chen: (pauses, assumes a confident air) and says: "If a tree falls in a forest and no-one is there ...."

Matrix Lesson 62

Never say: "That's a board question!"

At every Matrix Conference, one participant will lean back, assume the professorial demeanor and tell the presenting resident that the particular problem presented will be the basis of a "board question." In days past this was a helpful comment. Currently, the extended opportunities to pass the board examinations have lessened the impact of these comments.

The board exams serve a valuable purpose in surgery - tax deductible travel to new cities. Propriety prevents me from discussing the only other time one will plunk down a few hundred dollars to go to a hotel room with a stranger and work up a sweat!

The surgical board exam is made up of a written and an oral portion. Over the years a great mystique has been built up around these exams. Stories of exams are passed on from generation to generation forming a great oral surgical tradition.

A surgeon never forgets the board exam. (Nor does he ever forget his first St. Pauli girl.)

The second part of the board exam is an oral examination. The examination team travels to major United States cities, varying the locations year by year. The candidate arrives and goes from hotel room to hotel room guided by a piece of paper. He is interviewed by a pair of surgeons. One surgeon is a member of the board, and one is a local expert. These examinations, at last report, have become kinder and gentler. Gone are the blustery days of verbal harangues, stress interviews and surgical badgering.

The board has truly gotten in touch with its inner feelings and has recognized that surgeons need a warm and nurturing environment that pays full respect to their self-esteem, psychosocial development and ethno-cultural background to produce a warm and caring individual who recycles.

Because the board exam is so important to surgeons, many remember the questions which were asked. Many of these questions are the same from year to year.

There are two reasons for this:

■ The principles of clinical surgery do not change that much.

Human biology, in my lifetime, will probably not evolve to the point of changing some basic medical concepts. It took man four million years to evolve to his current state of physiology, so at least for the press run of this book, those principles will not change. The questions posed about those principles, therefore, will not change.

■ The examiners for the board do not change that much.

The men of the board are a somewhat static crew. None has ever been on Leno. If the rank and file of surgery are congressmen, these guys are senators. They seem to appear year after year. They are a serious lot, often wearing corduroy sportscoats in August.

"... the boards are important, but not more important than practical principles of surgery."

This fact, plus the intensity of the examination process causes many surgeons to remember the questions which they were asked. As the years go by, when a point of discussion comes up and a question is posed, the frequent refrain thus becomes: THAT'S A BOARD QUESTION!

The problem is that those questions usually do not form part of the day-to-day practice of surgery. They are not germane to present practice, and are, by and large, not useful to the working surgeon. To be fair, although some questions may relate to safe principles of managing common diseases, a larger number may relate to uncommon circumstances surrounding uncommon diseases.

In addition to this, the answer - time-honored as it is - may be wrong or at best not up-to-date. Imagine biliary questions during the introduction of laparoscopic cholecystectomy, regarded by some in its early devlopment as surgical adventurism. Imagine questions about low rectal lesions as the candidate wrestles with the use of stapling devices against the perceived surgical conservatism of the examiner. In these situations, the expected and acceptable board answer may, in fact, be the *wrong* answer.

It is this dichotomy between daily practice and board expectation that has led to two developments: the formulation of Matrix Lesson #62 and the policy of the board to fail to invite me to examine for them.

As Assistant Editor of our surgical newsletter, I wrote a satirical column called "Ask Professor Ted." Troubled surgeons of the nineteen nineties wrote letters to none other than Professor Theodor Billroth, seeking his advice and counsel. Across the ages Professor Ted answered these letters.

One particular letter bears review with reference to Matrix Lesson #62:

Dear Professor Ted:
I have failed the surgical board exams two times. Any pointers?
(Signed) Failed in Philly.

Dear Abject Failure:
As I tell all of my studenten, there is only one other time in a man's life when he will plunk down $500 in order to go to a hotel room with a strange person!

As a board examiner, I offer the following advice:

- Stay up the entire night before the exam.
- Wear a blue blazer - the official blazer of the surgical academic.
- Go to a shoe store and get a pair of "board shoes." The shoe salesman will know what you want. These are 30# wing-tip shoes designed by a cobbler in Philadelphia. (Incidentally, these can be bronzed after the exam and your family can put them in your childhood dresser next to your baby shoes.)
- Eat a large breakfast the morning of the exam. I prefer spiegeleier mit shinken, bratwurst covered with melted Muenster, two water bagels, a sachertort, two trips to the "endless blintz tray" and a Ramos fizz. This meal is essential for inducing the torpid state consistent with the netherworld the examinee is about to enter.
- Practice cordiality. No high-fünfs on entering the room.
- Practice the examinee's stance - seated relaxed, hands folded, jacket unbuttoned.
- Always check your inside coat pocket! A telltale cocktail napkin, or a brochure from the Pink Cat Escort Service is an automatic fail.

- Listen carefully to the examiner. As he leans forward in an ever-increasing frenzy of professorial nonsense, offer him a tic-tac^{TM}, or in extreme cases, an altoid^{TM}.
- Never void before the exam. A full bladder, stressed to the absolute limit of receptive relaxation is a great stimulus for short to-the-point-answers.
- Pace your responses. As they say in professional sports, learn clock management.
- Never respond to any of the following questions:
  a) Who is your chief?
  b) Where did you say you were from?
  c) See you next year!
- Leave the room bowing and walking backwards.

Sincerely, Professor Ted.

Matrix lesson #62 teaches us that the boards are important, but not more important than practical principles of surgery. There should be no difference between the answer to a board question and what a surgeon would do in the best interests of his patient.

Matrix Lesson 63

A resident educates himself*

Every resident and intern should be familiar with the scene in the *Paper Chase* (I forget if it was in the movie, the series or the book), in which Professor Kingsfield responds to a question from a first year law student about the material to be covered in his contracts class.

The Professor replies: "You teach yourself the law. I will teach you how to think like a lawyer."

I have yet to find a better synopsis of the essence of medical education. The surgical resident teaches himself surgery. The Matrix Conference teaches him how to *think* like a surgeon.

* I use the term "himself" in the aggregate pre-feminist contextual sense.

Note to residents: have no illusions about who is ultimately responsible for your surgical education. You are!

The education of the surgical resident is self-driven. The resident educates himself. It makes no difference who is the chief. It makes no difference that the research department has been awarded a $5 million NIH grant to study rat bladders. The bells and whistles in the operating theater mean nothing. The staff's curricula vitae (see Matrix Lesson #85) mean even less. None of these educate the resident.

Although it was known to some, it was one of the great revelations of my life when I realized that resident education is uniformly the lowest priority of any department of surgery. It makes no difference if that department is enclosed by the ivy walls of the East Coast, or the rhododendral walls of the West Coast.

The reason for this is quite simple. Medical education is a cost-loser in a cost-conscious world. The mission statement may list patient care, research and education as its tripartite goals, but the accountants and spreadsheet-makers pay attention to only the first two.

Education generates no income. Despite the lip service, the feigned dedication, the overwhelming concern and the fealty paid to resident education, it is #456 on the departmental priority list (#455 is emeritus parking).

"Note to residents: have no illusions about who is ultimately responsible for your surgical education. You are!"

"Resident education" is a lot like "national security" - an emotional term that inspires but may not deliver. The amazing thing is that, for the dedicated resident, it makes no difference. What the resident needs to educate himself is simple and is available in many venues:

■ A burning need to learn surgery and an insatiable appetite for surgical knowledge.

Notice I refer to a *need* to learn surgery, not just a *desire*. This semantic difference will not be lost on the literate reader. During his education, and hopefully throughout his career, this need is never totally fulfilled. It separates training from education. Many surgeons are trained. Only a few are educated.

■ A good medical library open 24 hours a day with free copying and internet privileges.

Medical libraries in teaching hospitals should always be open. We pay for retreats and focus groups. We pay for meetings and a multiplicity of worthless surgical endeavors. We airlift semi-embalmed professors across the continent and put them up in fancy hotels. Take that money and pump it into the medical library so I can ask the intern to present a brief biographical vignette in German in the morning about Frau Thérèse Heller.

■ A hospital with sick people in it.

The accent here is on sick people.

■ A department of surgery.

I am not referring to the bureaucratically-layered, administratively concretized prototypes of the mega-department. I am talking about a group of people who are committed to surgical education and who will devote time to the residents.

This department needs an administrative secretary assigned to the residents. When the history of surgery is written, resident-assigned secretaries and program co-ordinators will, in the long run, be better surgical educators than most professors.

Working surgeons.

In order to master surgery, residents need to be associated with working surgeons. Professors are great - they can opine on the differences between phlebothrombosis and thrombophlebitis. But the residents need a surgeon who can show them how to safely take down a splenic flexure and how to dig out a diverticular mass.

Residents need surgeons who can show them how to talk to patients and their families. They need surgeons who can bridge the gap between theory and practicality. They need to work with the surgical lumpenproletariat - the people who run this great engine called clinical surgery.

The requirements for self-education are easy to come by in most programs. As the resident maps his four or five years, he will realize the validity of Matrix Lesson #63.

A resident educates himself.

Matrix Lesson 64

Never say: "We were dry when we closed."

All returns to the operating theater during the postoperative course are presented at the weekly Matrix Conference. The most frequent cause for re-operation in this setting is postoperative bleeding.

There are very few statements which deny the very existence of the state they try to describe. Whenever a surgeon says: "We were dry when we closed," he is, in fact, saying that we were *not* dry when we closed. The event he is discussing disproves the statement he just made.

"We were dry when we closed," is a standing semantic joke among surgeons. The surgeon may as well begin his presentation with: "A priest, a rabbi and a minister were in an airplane ..." WWDWWC usually precedes a litany of self-rebuke most often following a re-exploration for bleeding usually in the wee hours of the morning.

It leads to a historical list of excuses (see *Gordon's Lexicon of Surgical Excuses* - in press). Those being:

- The dissection was extensive.
- The patient may have had a coagulopathy.
- It was a bloody case.
- The patient was on aspirin.

In a group or meeting setting, a not-so-silent groan can usually be heard when the presenting resident or surgeon speaks these words. The sentence has become part of the surgical lexicon.

What "we were dry when we closed" really signifies is:

- The resident closed and did not check for bleeding.
- I closed and missed the bleeding.
- The "oozing" described in the operative report crossed the hazy line into the field of "bleeding."

Lesson #64 implies that there is a better way to convey the message, that there did not seem to be any bleeding at the end of an operation. It implies that the surgeon made his best efforts to check for bleeding. Those efforts are never perfect.

> "Whenever a surgeon says: 'We were dry when we closed,' he is, in fact, saying that we were not dry when we closed."

It is surgically correct and semantically proper to use the following statements when describing a bleeding complication:

- "There did not seem to be a bleeding problem at the end of the procedure."

- "There were no signs of unusual bleeding at the end of the operation."
- "We examined all areas of dissection and found no bleeding."
- "I felt we had the bleeding controlled as we finished."

And finally, the most dramatic, refreshing and probably the most accurate statement:

- "We were *not* dry when we closed."

The phenomenon of being "dry when we closed" is aptly summarized in the country-western song "Don't The Girls All Get Prettier at Closing Time."*

This song, the anthem of the American Congress of Blood Banks, tells the tale of the lonely cowboy, desperate for female companionship. He seeks the perfect mate. At the beginning of the evening, his standards are high. He will not deviate from his standard of care - what a prudent cowboy would do in a similar situation.

As the evening progresses, it becomes obvious that his search is futile. He cannot meet his goals in the context of the time constraints of country-Western bar closure. Regrettably, he lowers his standards: "Ain't it funny. Ain't it strange. The way a man's opinions change."

The surgical analogy is clear. The weary surgeon confronted with bleeding is not the same cowboy he was when the case began. He may have lowered his standards for the ideal hemostatic field. His opinion of what a dry field is has changed. If these lyrics were to be re-written for surgery, the title would change to: "Don't The Fields all Get Drier at Closing Time."

---

* This song, written by Baker Knight, sung and popularized by Mickey Gilley, was #1 on the Country-Western charts during the first week of May, 1976. It is particularly appropriate that this be played during closure of cases in which bleeding is of concern. Many fine recordings of this song are available. My personal favorite is on the album "The Ultimate Mickey Gilley" on the Bransounds label.

If you use the proper statements listed above, your surgical techniques will no longer be suspect. Your honesty will be appreciated. Your attention to detail will not be questioned.

The alternative statements listed above are surgically correct and semantically appealing. They will not generate the knee-jerk suspicion of surgical sloppiness that arises every time a surgeon hears: "We were dry when we closed."

Matrix Lesson 65

Never refer to a patient as
an organ or as an operation

"There's a gallbladder in Room 3."
"The colon in 654 can eat."
"Send the appy home."
"See the hernia."

I would rather be labeled with the most heinously prejudicial name one could muster than be equated with a diseased organ.

I have read the sociologist-assigned-to-the-surgical-service-to-analyze-(courtesy of a huge grant)-surgical-insensitivity-study. I have reviewed the psychological profiles of surgeons. I have studied the inscrutable psychiatric assessments of the surgical mind. I have even read everything Richard Selzer has written. Nothing I have seen can ever explain the innate rudeness and total disregard for humanity that occurs every time a patient is referred to as a diseased organ.

This has nothing to do with surgery or medicine. It has nothing to do with the "hair shirt" or other fashionable psycho-babble. It has to with courtesy. It has to do with respect. It has to do with humanity. And, if I may quote my late mother, it has to do with manners.

I know of what I speak because, for a time, I was the "knee" in room 604. My father was the "aorta" in 506. My mother the "foot" in room 709. My son the "strabismus" in 203.

The tendency for surgeons, particularly surgical residents, to refer to patients as the diseased organ which they harbor, probably arose from the tendency of the surgical mind to categorize disease.

It is far easier to remember colon, gallbladder and hernia than it is to remember Marmelstein, O'Melmehey and Ploztckiweicsz. Nevertheless, there is a lot more to Marmelstein, O'Melmehey and Plot (whatever).

> "Nothing I have seen can ever explain the innate rudeness and total disregard for humanity that occurs every time a patient is referred to as a diseased organ."

There is, as we say, humanity - our raison d'etre as physicians. Referring to patients by their proper name shows a respect for the patient as an individual.

There was an immigrant patient who was a World War II veteran. He came to the United States in the 1920s, as so many others did, with a few dollars in his pocket. He learned English. He became successful. He volunteered and fought in World War II.

After the war, his success continued. He became a well-known philanthropist. He got ill and required a gastrectomy. The attending surgeon, himself a WW II veteran with a knowledge of the patient's war record, as well as philanthropic activity, was making rounds. As he left the room, he was asked by an enterprising intern, if "the gastrectomy needed any new orders." The surgeon (an ex-marine) stiffened. His neck veins distended and he shook. He took a deep breath. What followed, although softly spoken and dispassionately related, contained the energy expended during the famous George Brett home run pine tar incident.

"The *gastrectomy*," he began, "came to this country penniless. He wasn't some spoon-fed middle class dilettante coddled through medical school. The *gastrectomy* put three kids through college. He wasn't a freeloading recipient of the educational welfare state. The *gastrectomy* fought a war so kids like you could smoke dope and get laid in the sixties. The *gastrectomy* built a business from nothing and gave back to this city in a way far surpassing anything you will ever do."

The surgeon paused and said: "I suggest you call the *gastrectomy* by his proper name. When you refer to him as the *gastrectomy* you relegate his existence to a rote and thoughtless surgical footnote. It's a helluva lot more than that. You strip him of his humanity."

Then came the clincher: "Without a sense of humanity," he said, "you'll never be a good surgeon. More to the point, you'll never care for a patient of mine again." The lesson was learned. Matrix Lesson #65 was written in stone.

Matrix Lesson 66

Keep a surgical notebook

"Corollary #1 of Lesson #66: keep a complications notebook."

Few residents currently working have ever heard of a surgical notebook.

Before the days of Xerox™ machines, modems and computer services and well before the days of grants, there were four parts to a surgical residency: the patient, the library, the operating theater and the surgical notebook.

These notebooks were given to interns at the beginning of their training. They were blank leather-bound books. Each intern was required to draw in these books each of the operations in which he participated.

He was instructed to embellish these drawings with comments about the particular case. Artistic talent was not needed. What was needed was a desire to learn and to record. There was something wonderful about going from the operating theater to the notebook, thinking through the case and recording it while fresh in the mind.

I would show you my notebook, but it is in the Smithsonian.

At the end of five years, each finishing resident would have a complete notebook of many operations annotated, amended and embellished by his own growing surgical knowledge. It was better than any text. It was one of the grand traditions of surgical education.

The surgical notebook should be revived.

The total cost for a thirty-five-member surgical residency would be about $200.00. These notebooks would form the basis for discussions with attending surgeons, as the residents record in their own hand and with their own perception what they had seen. The notebook grows and takes on a life of its own as they are amended, added to, annotated and revised.

In addition to the operative notebook should be a complications notebook. This book would be a compilation of each complication the intern or resident presented. These should also be annotated and should contain line drawings, references and comments.

How could one ever forget the nuances of a complication after so carefully recording it? Since surgical complications occur in set patterns (wound problems, anastomotic problems, bleeding problems, etc.), this notebook will serve as a reference tool throughout the year.

In a more sedate time, services often competed to see which service could produce the best notebook by the end of the academic year.

Such notebooks were also a time-saver since complications of a similar type occur frequently during the year. The classic work, *Surgical Complications* by Artz and Hardy began, I am told, with an industrious intern making a surgical complications notebook!

If a resident dedicates himself to a surgical complications notebook, he will leave a permanent testimony to the dispassionate assessment of his professional mistakes. It is his only shot at surgical immortality, for a book speaks through the ages.

The concept and tradition of the notebooks serve another purpose; it perpetuates and codifies the surgeon who created it. When a surgeon dies, what will be left? A meager pension plan, a modest home, a few shares of some worthless biotechnical stock. His wife will soon forget him, saving her energies for her new husband! His children will barely remember the haggard shell who missed every family affair because, as he so often mumbled, he had been "bumped"!

But, thanks to Matrix Lesson #66, the memory of the surgeon, through the surgical notebook, will last forever.

Matrix
Lesson 67

The first rule of the operating room
visitor is: get permission from the
operating surgeon *before* speaking

Operating theaters are busy places. Anesthesiologists, operating theater technicians, all strata of nursing administration, surgeons, residents, visitors and colleagues may all enter.

Going from room to room is part of the camaraderie and dare I use an outmoded medical word, "fun"* of being a surgeon: seeing the variety of cases being done; the varying pathology; the skills or lack thereof of one's colleagues; the displayed X-rays; and the resident involvement.

---

* Fun is a concept rapidly disappearing from clinical medicine today. All of our many detractors do their best to eliminate fun from our profession. To a degree, observing and analyzing the lessons presented in this book will revive a spirit of fun. As my Dad always said: "You have to have fun at work!"

How could anyone become anything other than a surgeon after spending a day in a set of busy operating suites? Visiting these rooms naturally leads to conversation. Here is where the very valuable Matrix Lesson #67 applies.

Late in my own residency, I was in a tight operative spot. The patient was not doing well; nor was I. A fellow resident entered the room, peered over the drapes, surveyed the situation and proclaimed: "Can you believe those ... Red Sox!"

It is rude and improper to engage in conversation with the operating team without first checking with the operating surgeon. This includes nurses and anesthesiologists.

The contradiction here is that most of the time, when cases go well, the operating theater takes on a social tone. This is as it should be, as it is an essential element of the team approach to surgery. Arising from that social tone, however, is an informality that lends itself to spontaneous conversation.

It must also be remembered that the only one really on the line during the case (besides the patient) is the operating surgeon. He is surgically responsible for what happens. To honor and to appreciate that responsibility, one should check with him before speaking to him or to members of the surgical team: "Dr. Gordon. May I speak?"

"It is rude and improper to engage in conversation with the operating team without first checking with the operating surgeon."

It is annoying and may even be disrupting to hear, as one is deep in the pelvis looking for the ureter, as beads of sweat form on the forehead, as the myriad details of the case race through the surgeon's mind to hear the following snippets: "Mindy, did you get lunch relief?" "As Freud said: 'Sometimes a hot dog is just a hot dog'." "I went but the food was *dreck*!" "If I don't cover the spread, they'll fit me for concrete shoes!"

The proper demeanor for the operating theater visitor is simple: enter the room. Say "Dr. Gordon, may I speak with Dr. Czyzz for a minute?" The response will either be "Yes," "Not now," or "thanks for observing Matrix Lesson #67; come back in a few minutes."

Matrix Lesson 68

The scrub suit is the garment of enlightenment

How does the world envision a doctor? Look to print and to film to conjure up the spirit of medicine. Watch television. Stroll through a medical center. The image of the doctor is not the image of a suit behind a desk asking about a family history of licorice addiction.

The image of a doctor is that of a tousled sleep-deprived, coffee-drinking physician who is clothed in a white coat over scrub suit.

The scrub suit is the uniform of the working physician. The scrub suit is the garment identifying that doctor as part of the grand lineage of surgeons. All surgeons wear scrub suits. It is a distinguishing garment unlike the double-breasted French-cut 38 long (pre-shrunk). The scrub suit is the uniform of the worker. The scrub suit is the uniform of the healer. The scrub suit is the uniform of the doctor who is tackling pathology with his own body and soul. It is the uniform of the fully committed, the disciplined and (I can hear the groans in the department of medicine) the brave. It is the uniform of the medical marine!

Disregard all hospital rules regarding the wearing of scrub suits. Wear them all around the hospital. Wear them on the way to work. Wear them to committee meetings, in the staff lounge, in the coffee shop. Wear them at local restaurants adjacent to the hospital. You have earned the right to wear them, so wear them!

The scrub suit is the garment of the educated, the garment of the surgeon, the garment of medical enlightenment! I can prove this. Go to any hospital between 18:00 Hrs. and 19:00 Hrs. Go to the surgeon's dressing area and what will one see? One will see legions of non-surgeons changing into scrub suits.

It is as if, at nightfall, they can realize their deepest dreams and aspirations - to wear the suit that is the hallmark of medical intelligence. To be, even if just in the darkness of the medical center night, a surgeon. They sneak down there, shed their daytime garments and for the next twelve hours revel in the fact that they can wear a scrub suit.

"Disregard all hospital rules regarding the wearing of scrub suits."

As in some B vampire movie, to their dismay, when the sun rises, they must return to their previous state, shed the garments they so desperately want to wear, and resume their own tasks. Why do they do this? They do it because they understand the principles behind Matrix Lesson #68.

Matrix
Lesson 69

A $500 fine or six months in jail for
every exclamation point or question
mark found in the progress notes

The patient had an appendectomy last year!!!
Where is the report of the barium enema?
The V-Q scan was never performed!!!
Pt. given albumin! Why????
The CAT scan report is not available!!!
Where is the study???
K = 6.7!!!
Why was this not done?

Proper punctuation is important to the grammarian
and to the surgeon. Progress notes should be carefully
worded and free of spelling errors. These notations should
be properly punctuated.

There are, however, two punctuation marks that have
no place in the medical progress notes. The progress

notes are for the recordation of the progress of the patient and the thought processes of the doctor as he tries to figure out what is wrong. They are also the place to dispassionately comment on the patient's progress.

"Exclamation points have no place in the medical record."

The progress notes are not for editorializing, pontificating or musing. Which brings us to the role of certain punctuation marks. Punctuation marks developed during early Medieval times as a means of communication. The scribe who wrote the text could not verbally communicate with the reader. He therefore, had to come up with something to communicate the message of a prayer or a psalm. Part of that communication was to convey intensity, query, emphasis or excitement. Punctuation was born.

There is no need for such punctuation in a medical record, unless you are not on speaking terms with the other consultants. The dash, the semicolon and the colon (a surgically proper name for a punctuation mark) have their own subtext. They are appropriate for surgical progress notes because they are emotionally neutral punctuation marks. But the exclamation point and the question mark signify medical editorialization or pontification.

The exclamation point is used by those surgeons who, because they cannot effectively communicate verbally, act out in the chart. By using the exclamation point, they shout and exclaim into the medical netherworld - that abyss into which we all occasionally shout about the imponderables of medicine.

Most of us do this on our own in the privacy of our minds. Some, unfortunately, do it in the chart. These physicians clutter the medical record with such goodies as: "I ordered this last week!" or "This is yesterday's K+!" Or, my favorite: "The patient had a hysterectomy!"

There is no place in the medical record for a sudden impassioned or emphatic utterance - the specific situation requiring an exclamation point.

The exclamation point should be used for verbal exclamatory sentences or for verbal commands. They are fine on rounds, in a conference, or during discussions.

Exclamation points have no place in the medical record.

The proscribed resident punishment for use of the exclamation point is:

- Prepare a brief biographical vignette of Charles Bingham Penrose.
- Explain the difference between thrombophlebitis and phlebothrombosis.
- Discuss pseudo-pseudo-pseudo hyperparathyroidism.
- An Addisonian male has a nasogastric tube in for three days. He is on a potassium-lowering diuretic. He is a left-handed poly-dipsic, hypophosphatemic vegetarian from the Goiter Belt. What is the sodium content per liter of his urine?
- According to the 1993 Morbidity and Mortality weekly, how many people in the United States committed suicide because of intractable pruritis ani?

After completing one of these assignments, exclamation points will disappear from the records.

Which leads us to a discussion of the question mark in the medical record. The medical record, for those who use it and write in it, is as of this writing an *inanimate object*. It cannot speak. Therefore, it cannot answer a question. We now have the situation in which grown men and women are asking an inanimate object a question. Only on the psychiatry service could we find such individuals.

Why then are questions placed in it? (This is a book, not a medical record, so I can use the question mark here.) Physicians who ask questions in the medical record are the descendants of the ancient medical philosophers who used to hang around the oracles in ancient Greece.

"Using question marks in the medical record is a great link to our philosophical past, but serves no current purpose."

Why is he jaundiced? Why is the hematocrit 25%? Why is the leg cool and pulseless? Who is being asked? Random questions appear in the record and are tossed out into the abyss of the medical center. Whom is the physician addressing? If one knows the answer, how should it be framed and to whom should it be delivered?

Staring into the medical record-oracle, these physicians place their questions and then leave. Nature is now out of balance - a misdirected unanswered question has appeared. It is left hanging.

Using question marks in the medical record is a great link to our philosophical past, but serves no current purpose.

If one has a question, ask it verbally and to the proper party. Use the chart notes for reliable observations, recommendations and facts.

Matrix Lesson 70

Beware the accent

The dynamic of the Matrix Conference is the dynamic of the lively debate over medical principle. The arguments, verbal jousting and comments represent the great oral tradition of the conference. People speak. The audience listens carefully.

Part of the fun of listening at the Matrix Conference is to see if one can detect place of birth, education or locale by noting the accent or speech habits of the speaker.

It has always amazed me how the son of a South Boston Irish immigrant, after attending Harvard and visiting various European clinics can wind up with a British accent. I am stupefied when the son of Sophie and Phil Klemsciewiecziecz winds up talking like one of the Cabots of Beacon Hill.

I have observed this illogical accent acquisition many times in my career. Otherwise sane people, all of a sudden, at a particular point in their career, begin to sound as if they are the Third Earl of Southfield!

These are the children of the *dese*, *dem* and *dose*; the children of Revere (the city not the Paul), the first generation descendants of people from County Cork, the sons and daughters of people from Minsk.

A red flag is raised when the accent does not comport with the place of birth.

Perhaps it was the six-hour layover at Heathrow. Perhaps Masterpiece Theater has dominated his life. Maybe he's a Benny Hill fan. Whatever it is, the gentrified British accent slowly appears. The quizzical look from a former associate is the most dramatic tip-off to the false accent. The newly acquired accent bespeaks an underlying insincerity. If genuine, the accent may, to some degree, influence the interpretation of what is said. Anything stated in a British accent, for example, is always true. Anything with a French accent is always suspect. Anything with a Southern accent is always humorous. Anything with a Texas accent is interesting and finally, anything said with a Chicago accent is eminently practical.

A special note about one particular word - *centimeter*. This word should be pronounced as if it were sentimeter, i.e. with a short e. It should be pronounced the same way cent is pronounced in "one red cent" or "two cents plain." The hallmark of the fake accent is the pronunciation of centimeter as santimeter (with a droning endlessly accented short a).

"A red flag is raised when the accent does not comport with the place of birth."

Why does this happen? It happens, near as I can figure, when your adjusted gross income exceeds $200,000 per year. I have never met a person making less than $200,000 per year who said santimeter. I have never met a person making more who did not say santimeter.

Somehow, through the surgical cortex, adjusted gross income triggers a linguistic response to mispronounce this word and to create a fake accent.

When I hear a surgeon pronounce this unit of measurement in this manner, I smile and ask the name of his accountant.

Most people with these affected accents talk just like you and me when awakened from a sound sleep. Try it. Call them at 2AM. It takes anywhere from three to five seconds for the fake accent to kick in.

Matrix Lesson 71

Resident involvement in an operation is earned

"Corollary #1 of Lesson #71: that involvement is delineated and explained before the operation begins."

Who "does" a case? What does "doing" a case mean?

There is wide variability across the country in resident involvement in surgical procedures. There is even more variability among the attitudes of attending surgeons towards that involvement. This variability reflects different philosophies of how surgery is taught in the operating theater.

The philosophies of operative involvement fall into three general categories:

■ Philosophy #1. The resident does nothing.

The resident assists an experienced surgeon who instructs him, educates him and intellectually challenges him.

The resident is lucky to be there. He is lucky to be able to sit at the foot of the master. He basks in the brilliance of the attending surgeon.

■ Philosophy #2. The resident does everything.

The resident is assisted by a capable surgeon who neither teaches him anything about the disease state, nor instructs him on his operative technique. The resident is the surgeon. The attending is an automaton.

■ Philosophy #3. The resident is *awarded* graduated operative responsibility, based on an interplay of talent, level, interest and knowledge.

The attending surgeon carefully controls the case. The surgeon never lets the resident forget that resident operative responsibility is earned. It is earned by demonstrating a kaleidoscopic knowledge of the patient, the operation and the disease state being addressed

Matrix Lesson #71 is founded on Philosophy #3.

An operation is not an isolated event. It is a continuum. Unfortunately, some residents demonstrate an increasing tendency to view the operation as a stand-alone event. This view developed because of the rise of outpatient work-ups and the concept of the AM admit.

Residents see the "operation" but do not see the myriad details and plans that led up to the operation. Sometimes, they do not see the follow-up after the operation.

The job of the legitimate surgical educator is to combat this denigration of surgical activity by making sure that resident operative responsibility is earned. It is earned by the resident who has a global view of the surgical procedure. It is earned by those residents who demonstrate a knowledge of the patient, the procedure and the disease. Awarding surgical responsibility without demanding such knowledge sells the resident short. In a greater sense, it sells short the discipline of surgery.

Which gets us to corollary #1 of Lesson #71.

Resident responsibility must be clarified and delineated *before* the procedure begins.

I have frequently observed the delicate interplay between eager resident and attending staff just prior to the case. In many instances it is akin to a junior-high dating situation. Both parties want to be there, but they are unsure as to what is expected of them.

There is a palpable uneasiness as the resident's desire to operate colors his actions. A ritual dance follows, not unlike those National Geographic specials on the mating habits of the pheasant. If the delineation of operative responsibility has not been made clear, resident and attending dance around the table, jockey for position, make moves with the drapes and reach for instruments. It is as if they are participating in a bizarre ceremony. It is a hilarious display of the mutual reluctance to discuss a vital topic - resident responsibility and the relative comfort of the attending surgeon with that responsibility.

All of this can be eliminated if the lines of responsibility are discussed beforehand.

To the residents: ask the question: "What is my role in this procedure?" To the attending surgeon: tell the resident what his role will be. For example: "I'll let you open and assess. Then you'll assist me." "You open and assess, take down the right colon and I'll let you go as far as I think you should." "You'll be assisting me on this case. If you're unhappy with that, get someone else in here."

The most important element of an operation is neither the resident's education nor the attending's allegiance to surgical education. The most important element is the obligation to get the case done with the maximum safety using the maximum surgical expertise available.

Participatory surgical education is the fallout of this obligation.

Matrix Lesson 72

Learn the art of taxis

I am a master of taxis.
I was taught by a master of taxis.
Taxis is an art form.
Take impressionism.
Give me taxis.
Learn it. Master it. Never forget it.

Most surgeons feel that the way to reduce an incarcerated groin hernia is to press on it - hard. To a large degree, this is what they have been taught. It certainly is what many emergency room physicians have been taught. They would frequently call me and say that they tried to reduce the hernia and could not.

The reason they could not reduce the hernia is that they do not understand the art of taxis.

I usually reduce these hernias easily because I practice taxis - the art of hernia reduction.

Taxis relies on a working knowledge of groin anatomy, an understanding of the dynamics of the internal inguinal ring and a further understanding of the anatomy and physiology of the mechanics of incarceration.

"Taxis will be increasingly important in our evolving healthcare system. Within five years it will probably be the only treatment allowable for incarcerated hernias."

Taxis is not properly taught in surgical education programs today. Walk up to any young professor of surgery, look him in the eye and say "taxis" and undoubtedly the first thing he will think of is H & R Block!

To quote one of my boyhood idols, the Prussian surgeon, Dr. Sultan: "Taxis is performed by firmly grasping and compressing the region of the neck of the hernial sac with the left hand and then exerting a uniform and constant pressure upon the entire hernial tumor with the right hand, taking care not to press the hernia toward, but rather to draw it away from the abdomen."*

As I wander through the emergency room, I see residents and some attendings attempting to reduce hernias by merely pressing on them. There is grunting by the resident and by the patient. There is groaning by

* *Atlas and Epitome of Abdominal Hernias.* Dr. Georg Sultan. First Assistant in the Surgical Clinic in Gottingen, Prussia. Edited by William B. Coley, M.D. Clinical Lecturer in Surgery, Columbia University, Assistant Surgeon to the Hospital for Ruptured and Crippled, New York City. Philadelphia and London: W.B. Saunders & Company, 1902.

the resident and the patient. Beads of sweat form on the resident's brow. Beads of sweat form on the patient's brow as an increasing number of physicians wander by and press firmly on his groin.

Frustration borne of anatomic ignorance follows! A call to the operating theater is made. There is more to reducing a hernia than by pushing on it.

Using taxis does three things:

- Taxis reduces the hernia.
- Taxis gets me back to sleep.
- Taxis allows me to perform the operation at the convenience of the patient and at my convenience.

Taxis will be increasingly important in our evolving healthcare system. Within five years it will probably be the only treatment allowable for incarcerated hernias. Gatekeepers will have to learn it, since access to surgeons will only be for taxis failures.

Dr. Sultan's 1902 text on taxis will again be the gold standard of hernia treatment.

The classic taxis story in our office happened in the wee hours one morning several years ago. After successfully reducing a hernia that the emergency room physician and several residents could not reduce, I looked at the resident and said: "Taxis!"

"Taxes!" the patient shouted. "All you doctors ever think about is money!"

Matrix Lesson 73

Study and master accordionology or take the colonoscopic estimate of a lesion's location with a 6kg grain of salt

---

Several surgical complications may arise if the surgeon is confronted with a colon lesion far away from the site described by the referring gastroenterologist. When these complications are discussed at the Matrix Conference, the discussion usually gets around to the emerging field of accordionology.

I have a great deal of respect for our gastroenterologic colleagues. They are a bright and earnest crew who seem to know all about sprue. Some are expert colonoscopists. However, despite their expertise, they know very little about accordionology - that branch of physiology which studies the physics of the accordion.

The accordion, a much maligned instrument, must be studied in detail by the surgeon who hopes to excel at colon surgery. In colonic terms, accordionology governs the anatomy and physiology of the colonoscoped colon. It governs the tendency of the colon to telescope onto the colonoscope.

Surgeons must be students of accordionology since their operations rely on the level and location of the colon lesion. Assessing the level of the lesion is crucial to the planning and safe performance of the operation. This is why, to a great degree, the success of colon surgery relies on the same things that successful restaurant planning relies on - location, location, location!

Gastroenterologists, on the other hand, just dabble in accordionology. They know the discipline exists, but will never have to make a crucial decision based on its tenets. They are to colon surgery what a football fan is to a football player.

Gastroenterologists are dilettantes of accordionology. Surgeons are board-certified accordionologists.

"Surgeons must be students of accordionology since their operations rely on the level and location of the colon lesion."

Since many surgeons do not perform their own colonoscopy, they may frequently be in a position of having to rely on the gastroenterologist for an assessment of the level of the colon lesion.

Which brings us to the first principle of surgical accordionology - the surgeon should not get into the habit of rotely relying on the gastroenterologist's estimated colonoscopic location of the lesion as a guide to his surgery.

Because of the physics of accordionology, the 25cm lesion can be anywhere from 6cm to 40cm. The 6cm lesion can be mid-sigmoid. The splenic flexure can become the hepatic flexure. The hepatic flexure can become the splenic flexure.

The fundamental principles of accordionology place the surgeon in a delicate situation when it comes to interacting with the gastroenterologist. If one wants to see a steady stream of referrals, one cannot be candid. One must be delicate. One must be sensitive to the psychosocial structure of the gastroenterologist's existence.

My answer to the problem is as brilliant as it is delicate and unique. I tell the patient that I am getting a special X-ray that will help clean out their colon prior to surgery. I order a water-soluble contrast enema for the day prior to surgery. The colon is cleaned. The referring doctor is impressed by my unique approach. I get to see the actual level of the lesion.

I understand accordionology. I now plan my operation.

Oh, I can hear the academic purists groaning now - "Dr. G got snookered once in 1981 and now he's subjecting his patients to 'unnecessary' tests."

My friends, e-mail me at MatrixPearls@Gmail.com after the low anterior resection for the "mid-descending" colon lesion. Call me after the famous "intra-operative colonoscopic lesion hunt." Call me after the left colectomy through the right subcostal incision. Call me when you find no lesion. Call me again after you have mastered accordionology.

Matrix Lesson 74

Nobody wants to be Scrooge

"Corollary #1 of Lesson #74: use the social history to justify an overnight stay."

"Corollary #2 of Lesson #74: don't let cost-containment become care-containment."

The #16 bus in Los Angeles runs East and West from downtown to the West side of town. The bus route courses through many neighborhoods. It services several medical centers. In the late afternoon on any given day, several elderly men will be sitting in the long back seat up against the back wall of the bus. This location allows them to stretch out and to shift position without inconveniencing fellow public transportation users.

If one studies their faces, one will see a look of concern. They will appear uncomfortable as they shift from side to side. Should the bus come to an abrupt halt, or even more revealing, hit a pot hole, they will, in unison yell "Oy!" or "Ow-w-w" or "Aie-e-e-e!"

These are the men who have had outpatient hernia repairs. These are the men who have been sent home on the afternoon of their surgery. These are men whose groins have been anatomically re-arranged just hours before this ride. These are the men whose spermatic vessels have been moved and whose scrota have been traumatized by inquisitive surgical interns. These are men who face an evening at home, walking back and forth from the television chair to the ice tray. Why are these men on the #16 bus rather than in a hospital room?

The answer is cost-containment - the byword of medical economics for the last twenty years. Cut costs by "streamlining" care. Cut costs by "judicious use of laboratory tests." Cut costs by keeping hospitalizations to a "minimum." Nowhere is this more obvious than with outpatient surgery. Patients who normally would have been hospitalized are sent home in the name of cost savings.

Often, the concerned surgeon will realize that some of these patients are truly better served by admitting them to the hospital for one night. With many insurance plans and in many hospitals, however, this is difficult to justify on a purely medical basis. On a practical, common sense and humanitarian basis however, it is rather easy to justify.

The surgeon is in the middle. He is there to provide care, not to deny care. He does not want to be Scrooge. He does not want *care-containment*. What parts of the medical record can we use to justify a common sense decision?

The physician must be creative with his use of the medical history. The most fertile area for this creativity lies in the social history. Many facts may be used to support an overnight admission. Their wording is crucial.

They must be worded in terms that make it impossible for anyone with a beating heart to send the patient home.

For example:

■   "This is an elderly male recently operated upon. He lives alone and must go up eight flights of stairs to return to his one-room cold-water flat. Admission tonight is medically indicated since he cannot negotiate these steps." This is always approved.

■   "The World War II veteran has no means of transportation home. The taxi voucher is useless since no taxi driver will go into his neighborhood ..." or

■   "This patient suffered a premature ventricular contraction during the operation. It is medically necessary that he be admitted tonight for observation." (Make sure PVC is singular.)

■   "This patient has severe prostatism and has trouble voiding. Admission is needed for incipient urinary retention." This is one of my favorites, since all elderly men have prostatism and, if you think about it, we are all in incipient urinary retention.

Matrix Lesson #74 puts the challenge of current healthcare restrictions in the name of cost-containment in a semantic, rather than a medical light. Concerned physicians must learn to rephrase the elements of the patient's disease in words that will retrospectively approve an admission.

Matrix Lesson #74 will prevent cost-containment from becoming care containment.

Matrix Lesson 75

Understand, study, analyze, appreciate and beware surgical hubris

---

The intrinsic dynamic of the Matrix Conference allows the audience to dissect the activity of the surgeon. Through a process of analysis and debate, question and answer, the mechanics of surgery are laid bare for review. Occasionally, a case is presented which represents a surgical complication that went unrecognized, despite being evident. Why does this happen?

The surgeon is often portrayed as a heroic figure. His work and his position are perceived by many as godlike. His presence in the middle of an emergency carries with it an aura of serious and focused intent.

Heroic action has always been the theme of great literature. Some of that literature shows us tragic heroes. The tragic hero becomes tragic through his own failings.

The surgeon may fail in the same manner. That failure may be due to a personal quality called *hubris*.

I have studied hubris since my first surgical rotation when I was confronted with the overweening pride of the over-educated, over-bearing surgical attending who had no insight into his own failures. This is the fertile ground in which hubris grows.

Hubris is the element of pride that, in its most basic definition, offends the gods. It offends them through a presumption of human greatness. It offends the gods by being insolent towards them.

"No surgeon is above their power which manifests itself in a hundred humbling ways on any surgical service."

I would sum up my knowledge of Greek tragedy by saying simply - don't mess with these gods, for they will put you on a fast-track to ruin.

The tragic Greek heroes of Greek literature passed through various stages.* There are definite analogies in surgical careers. *Olbos* was the initial stage of happiness and prosperity when the hero seemed blessed. This is the new attending surgeon. *Koros* described feelings of superiority. This is the insidious effect of experience on the maturing surgeon. *Hubris* followed. Hubris was the most lethal quality.

It is a dangerous physical and spiritual arrogance which preceded *ate* the pathetic blind fumbling against destiny, leading to ruin and desolation.

* Paraphrased from Emily Vermuele: "It's Not a Myth - They're Immortal" in *The Red Sox Reader*. Dan Riley. Ventura Arts, 1987.

Hubris was at the apex of tragic development. There are clear analogies in surgery. Surgeons who feel they are "above it all" or who feel they are protected from serious complications, because of their self-perceived brilliance, demonstrate hubris.

The surgeon afflicted with hubris is easy to spot. He's the one whose beeper mysteriously goes off when his complication is being discussed at the Matrix Conference.

As fickle and remorseful as the mythological gods were, so are the gods of surgery. No surgeon is above their power which manifests itself in a hundred humbling ways on any surgical service. Understanding hubris is the single most important ingredient to avoiding its devastating effects.

No surgeon, despite his innate talents, reputation, skill and accomplishments, is above an eternal appreciation of the power of surgical pathology, as well as its vagaries and its capricious nature.

When the surgeon acquires hubris, ruin follows usually at the expense of his patients. Hubris is surgery's way of keeping order in its ranks.

Matrix Lesson 76

The patient you want to remain at rest
will be rolled, cajoled and patrolled

"Obverse of Law #76: the patient
you want to be mobilized will be
neglected, rejected and
disaffected."

Certain operative-anatomic situations lead surgeons to insist that their postoperative patients lie still in bed: the difficult colectomy; the retroperitoneal tumor with extensive dissection; the delicate biliary reconstruction stented by a small T-tube.

These anatomic situations are burned into the surgeon's mind as he and his patient begin the postoperative period. They color his postoperative orders. Many surgeons prefer that such patients be limited in activity for twenty-four to forty-eight hours until things settle down.

Many surgeons feel that such immobilization may avoid some early postoperative problems: a drain dislodgement or a wound dehiscence.

On the other hand, there are certain patients whom the surgeon wants mobilized: the obese patient after a ruptured appendix; the chronic lung patient after an upper abdominal incision; the post-phlebitic patient after any operation.

Both approaches are an effort to avoid a postoperative complication. Both are clear and understandable desires of the surgeon.

Matrix Lesson #76 teaches us that the polar opposite of the surgeon's orders, wishes and desires will usually occur.

The patient you want lying in bed "gelling" will be mobilized, pummeled and shifted around immediately following the operation. Shortly after surgery, the respiratory technician, hitherto missing in action, will appear to roll, beat on and vibrate the patient. Various machines will be placed at the bedside. The room takes on the appearance of a deep-space training center.

A physical therapist fresh off of the taping of her own exercise video will appear to stretch and elongate the patient. The floor nurse will experience a sudden unbridled interest in mobilization orders. She will parade the patient around the room as the T-tube becomes coiled on the bathroom door. The carefully placed drain becomes intertwined with the television channel changer. The bladder catheter hooks itself on the bed-rail. The central line encircles the bedside water pitcher.

The occupational therapist, misdirected, enters the room and begins a welding session.

This all happens in the wee hours of the night as the surgeon is relaxing, confident that his orders are being implemented.

Now in the next room, is your patient for whom you ardently wish full and active mobilization. He is lying there like a plate of lox. Despite specific orders and entreaties, he is unattended. The respiratory rate is about four per minute and the tidal volume is forty cc. No-one comes into this patient's room for hours. He is a thrombogenic preparation. Tubes clot. Lines become disconnected. Intravenous lines run dry. Lenin gets better care.

I cannot explain the metaphysics behind Matrix Lesson #76. Deep in the recesses of the nursing psyche must be a force whose goal is to test the patient's physiologic reserve and to prove that the human body can withstand a variety of insults.

This same force challenges the coronary reserve of the surgeon. Fortunately there is an abundance of surgical coronary reserve and patient physiologic reserve.

Matrix Lesson 77

Full-time departments of surgery increase exponentially, independent of the economic climate in which they exist

Most Matrix Conference audiences are mixed audiences. This means that the attending level positions are comprised of both full-time surgeons, as well as private practice physicians with teaching obligations. Private practice surgeons have always been mystified by the continued growth of full-time departments of surgery. Matrix Lesson #77 explores this phenomenon.

We must remember the "begats" of the Old Testament. Jehosophat begat Nebuchedel who begat Cain who begat Sid, who begat Ethel. I, myself, have begat on at least two occasions.

As in the Bible, this same driving "begat" force causes professors to beget assistant professors who beget fellows who beget liaison nurses who beget nurse co-ordinators who beget departmental administrators who beget departmental co-ordinators who beget assistant departmental co-ordinators who beget liaisons to the assistant departmental co-ordinator ... on and on.

A department of biblical proportions results.

> "How is it that in a financially restrictive medical climate where every aspect of medical care is studied and analyzed that the numbers in a full-time division can proliferate?"

Full-time academic surgeons simply cannot function without a begotten entourage.

Despite an increasingly streamlined healthcare system; despite layoffs and cutbacks; despite the hue and cry over administrative costs, the begetting continues. The reason for this is interesting. The true professor feels that his insights and pronouncements are the crystalline light of pure surgical knowledge. This rare nectar; this most valuable entity simply should not be polluted with daily obligations.

How does one eliminate daily obligations and the mundane responsibilities of surgical life? Delegate them! The motto of the surgical professoriate is: *delegato ergo sum* (I delegate, therefore I am).

Fellows, residents, and other surgical *nachschleppers*, created under the guise of this educational motto, are there to shield the professor from the exigencies of daily surgical life, i.e. surgical work.

This allows the professor to:

- Plan the retreat.

The retreat is the hallmark of the full-time surgical department. This involves contracting with a "consulting firm." It means arranging "focus groups" and their "facilitators" to head the focus groups. This is laborious stuff since it involves a high level of delegation.

▦   Plan the sabbatical.

The sabbatical is the Lombardi Trophy of the professoriate. It is a paid vacation under the guise of deep-seated educational thought.

▦   Write the grant.

Under the new healthcare plan, this will not occupy much of the full-time surgeon's day, so he can concentrate on a more important task - the ultimate professorial task.

▦   Hire more people.

More people. More people. More people. The Government's answer to most problems is to throw more money at the problem. The professorial model is simply to change the unit of currency, i.e. to throw more fellows or junior attending surgeons at the problem.

Meanwhile, in the more accountable areas of the medical center, transportation workers, ward clerks and nurses are being laid off.

How is it that in a financially restrictive medical climate where every aspect of medical care is studied and analyzed, that the numbers in a full-time division can proliferate? It goes against economics. It goes against nature. It goes against common sense.

But this is the true genius of the professoriate - taking a seemingly contradictory and illogical phenomenon and justifying it.

Jesaph begat Mitabel who begat Dr. Flieber who is our new research associate who begat ...

Matrix Lesson 78

Learn to detort a sigmoid volvulus

Two facts conspire to make this an important lesson:

- We eat a low fiber diet. The largest growing segment of the population is the over-65 crowd.
- Our greatest form of exercise is moving the thumb over the 256 cable ready channel changer.

We now have a health threat for the millennium - millions of sigmoid volvuli!

Volvulus was the Roman god of Cramping. It was he, in the pantheon of Roman gods, whom Zeus called "Mr. Grumpy." The ancients had a tough choice - Volvulus or Ceres, the goddess of Whole Grain. Whomever they chose would govern their patterns of life. Edith Hamilton covered this already and I will not add to it.

"Sadly, the **proper treatment** of a **sigmoid volvulus** is rapidly becoming a **lost art** among surgical residents. It is an art ... an effortless **detorsion** of a sigmoid volvulus."

For embryological and dietary reasons, the sigmoid can twist on its mesentery. This can happen rapidly and dramatically. Its treatment requires sophisticated care. The Masai tribe in Africa has the largest stool weight per individual of any studied tribe. The Masai do not suffer sigmoid volvuli. Unfortunately, they all die by the age of fifty from wildebeast gorings as they squat in the bush. But that is not to be discussed here.

Our rapidly aging population assures that many sigmoid volvuli are headed to emergency rooms across the nation. Surgeons and surgical residents will be called upon to diagnose and to treat this increasingly common condition.

Sadly, the proper treatment of a sigmoid volvulus is rapidly becoming a lost art among surgical residents. It is an art. What is art anyway? To you it may be a Leroy Nieman retrospective. To me it is an effortless detorsion of a sigmoid volvulus.

Declining expertise in this area is most likely due to the general trend of getting away from the patient and getting involved in sophisticated studies. Detorting a volvulus requires a knowledge of the disease, a knowledge of the sigmoid and a desire to become an impresario with a rigid proctoscope.

I was taught by a master detorter. In his honor, I pass on this rich legacy. At every turn I am thwarted by ignorance of the disease, ignorance of sigmoid anatomy and a fascination with sophisticated studies.

I receive no grants from the NIH for passing on this information. The MacArthur foundation has not called. Bill and Melinda are not on hold. No-one has endowed a named chair in my honor. I have received no honorary degrees. No fund-raiser has had a poached salmon dinner for me, nor have I been solicited to chair any departments. Nevertheless, I fight on.

A rigid proctoscope manufactured in 1935, when properly used to detort a sigmoid volvulus, can do more than any GI fellow with a $7000 model x-6700 three-chip video-laser-CD-ROM triply-enhanced surround-sound colonoscope. Patient position, skill of detorsion, a knowledge of colonic physics, Charles' Perfect Gas Law, and an old scrub suit coupled with proper tube stenting, lead to effortless, successful detorsion of most volvuli.

The CAT scan of an 86-year-old patient with the sudden onset of abdominal distension, whose flat-film showed a bird beak pattern is interesting and stimulating.

But the detorsion of that volvulus based only on observation and proctoscopic skill is infinitely more satisfying.

Matrix
Lesson 79

Never answer an unattended,
ringing medical center telephone

The difference between a teenager and an adult is that when a phone rings the teenager desperately hopes that the call is for him.* Nowhere is this more vividly portrayed than with the unattended, ringing medical center telephone.

You are sitting and writing a progress note. You are standing at the nursing station. You are relaxing in the surgeons' lounge. You are walking down an empty hospital corridor. You are blissfully alone, involved in the work of the day. You pass a wall-mounted phone. It rings. You have paged no-one. It rings again. No-one is around to answer it. The nurses go about their work. Orderlies and residents walk by. The crucial decision is upon you.

---

* Variously attributed to Dorothy Parker, HL Mencken, Bennet Cerf and others.

I will give you the benefit of many tortuous excursions into the byways of a major medical center: *DO NOT ANSWER THAT PHONE!*

There were no phones on the Isle of Cos when Hippocrates went into practice. Galen did not have phones, nor did Paracelsus, Maimonides or Semmelweiss. Avicenna did not have a phone nor did Theophrastus Bombastus. If Fleming had had a phone in his lab we never would have heard of penicillin.

These men did their work unencumbered by the ringing telephone. If they had such phones and if they made the key error of answering them, they would be nameless physicians. They would not have made their great contributions. They would have had the medically frustrating experience of *phonus interruptus* - the interruption of the medical day with a disturbing unrelated phone call.

> "Your day is tough enough without absorbing the electronically transmitted ills of people you do not even know."

If that ringing phone is answered, there is a 99% chance that you will involve yourself with a most distasteful situation. *Never, ever answer that phone!*

If you do, you will become involved in some inextricably difficult hospital problem from which there is no exit. You will get involved in a cyclonic swirl of medical misery. *Do not answer that phone!*

That solitary ringing phone is a busy surgeon's worst nightmare. It is a ring which will destroy your day and will involve you in a course of events over which you have no control.

These calls fall into four general categories:

▤   The random call.

If the phone is answered, the voice (which, incidentally, never waits for a response) will say:

"Tell Bernie I'll take the Rams plus the points."
"Tell Power-ranger that the eagle flies at night."
"If Marie is there I'll come over and kill you."

The random call is the most innocuous and sometimes actually brightens a day. But this call is uncommon. One is more likely to get other types of calls.

▤   The family call.

The Carter family is extremely upset at the care Dad has been receiving. They call the nursing stations, the administrators and generally have a working knowledge of all of the phone extensions. One does not want to have anything to do with this family, even if it is the menial task of forwarding a message.

▤   The maintenance call.

Manny from plant operations is ready to flush the hoister valves, causing brown liquid to come out of several showers. He will only call once, and this is the extension he was given. He hangs up. After this call, clanking noises begin to arise from behind the walls. You are now in the middle of an ecologic-plumbing disaster.

▤   The lab call.

"Alice Grieg has a positive blood culture."
"The potassium is nine."
"There is tumor at the margin."

One does not want to hear this or be involved in these situations. Misery is attached to each statement as it comes through the phone. Your day is tough enough without absorbing the electronically transmitted ills of people you do not even know.

Ignoring the ringing phone is not an abrogation of medical responsibility. It is not an unfair or selfish act. It is not a violation of the Hippocratic Oath. Rather, avoiding those calls is a reasonable move in the middle of a busy day designed to facilitate that day.

Be vigilant - focus on your surgical duties and above all: *do not answer that phone!*

Matrix Lesson 80

Never take the fall for a consultant's error

Two complications were discussed at a recent Matrix Conference: a hepatic subcapsular bleed after attempted percutaneous drainage of a liver abscess; and a re-intubation following a re-intubation, which followed a re-intubation of a re-intubation after extubation by the anesthesiologist in the recovery room.

The residents' presentations were masterful. Their summaries were accurate. Their literature reviews were appropriate. Their list of Matrix points was complete. Their review of the studies showed the preparation and concern that went into their presentations. The discussions were heated. The discussions were interesting. But most importantly, the discussions were .... out of place.

Such discussions were out of place because the presenting physicians took the heat from the audience for *a management error that they did not commit.*

I remember those wonderful nineteen thirties Jimmy Cagney movies when Rocky took the wrap for Lefty so the gang could still function. Rocky got sent up the river while Lefty went to the Stork Club. But this was a medical meeting, not a movie. This was a Matrix Conference, not a sentencing hearing.

This was a conference designed to assess responsibility for medical errors and in so doing, to instruct those *who committed the error* on how to avoid that error in the future.

"Criticism should not be directed towards an attending or resident for someone else's errors."

Non-surgical consultants who cause or who are involved in complications which arise from their intervention should be responsible for discussing these problems. The surgical meeting is for complications arising from surgery performed, not from procedures performed by other physicians. Even though these procedures may be performed on surgical patients and may have surgical implications, the responsibility for discussing specific problems arising from them falls to the person who is most responsible.

If you talk the talk, you have to walk the walk. (I have no idea what this means but I saw this great movie on cable last week. Some weak-kneed non-combatant was relating all the battles he had been in as the eyes of his colleagues rolled upwards. I thought of that Matrix Conference.)

The interventional radiologist and the anesthesiologist have many interactions with the surgical service. These are independent physicians who perform their own procedures. They have their own departments. There is no logical reason why the attending surgeon or surgical resident should have to analyze, defend or discuss other consultant's errors of judgment or technique. That responsibility rests solely with the physician who performed the procedure.

While there is general educational benefit in discussing these problems, the Matrix Conference is not the place to do it. There is enough to discuss in the sphere of bona fide surgical complications without bringing in the complications of ancillary consultants.

The goal of the Matrix Conference is to analyze an error and to figure out, according to the principles of the discipline, how it happened and what might have been done to prevent it. That charge is impossible to carry out if the problem arises outside of the specialty of surgery.

Criticism should not be directed towards an attending or resident for someone else's errors. Surgery is tough enough and preparation for Matrix Conferences is tough enough without having to take the heat for a consultant's errors.

If the conference co-ordinator disagrees with Matrix Lesson #80, which is his right and privilege as a professor, a middle ground can often be reached by inviting the responsible physician to attend the meeting. At the end of the presentation he will comment on the problem.

The spirit of communal education and quality of care which permeates teaching hospitals will lead these physicians to gleefully and willingly accept that invitation.

Matrix Lesson 81

Use humor judiciously

"Corollary of Lesson #81:
humor is serious business."

One cannot be a surgeon without a sense of humor. On second thought, that is incorrect. One can be a surgeon without a sense of humor, but one can be a better surgeon with a sense of humor. Humor gives a surgeon humanity and insight into the human condition. At its most basic level there are essential elements of humor in surgery. Surgery is so far removed from anyone's sense of reality as to represent a contradiction. Contradiction is the essence of humor. Pointing out this contradiction is what humor in medicine is all about.

Several criteria must be met before a physician uses humor in a medical situation:

■   The physician must know the family or the patient.

Humor should never be used at the initial patient or family meetings. Patients and their families are coming to a surgeon, not trying to get tickets to the Improv.

■   The medical situation must not be urgent.

Despite sleep deprivation, high endorphin levels and the high tension inherent to the craft of medicine, humor is generally not used in urgent circumstances.

■   One must know when humor is failing.

I am reminded of the dying (in the show business sense) stand-up who keeps tapping the microphone and asking: "Is this on?"

There are great ethnic and societal differences in the response to humor. The surgeon must be culturally aware. For example, certain ethnic groups do not understand the comparison of a liver edge to an overdone potato kugel.

■   One must stop all attempts at humor after the first blank look.

Blank stares following attempts at humor are akin to blank stares during surgical board examinations. They are visual cues of instant humor failure.

Let's examine several recent humor-oriented surgical circumstances. Last week I was asked by Mrs. Sylvia Teitelbaum: "Doctor, how do you find Sidney today?" I know this family well. Sidney was recovering uneventfully. Ethnically and culturally I was in tune with Mrs. Teitelbaum. We were, as we say, on my block, *landsmen*.

As I reacted to this mundane question, I reasoned that it would be culturally and interpersonally appropriate to employ humor in my response. Taking care to observe appropriate attending rank behavior and being sensitive to any cross-cultural differences avoiding the insidious influences of ageism, I responded: "How do you think I find Sydney? I go down the corridor, take a left and go into room 7105! That's how I find Sidney today!" I pause. She laughs.

The humor strengthens the patient-family-surgeon bond.

On the other hand, we have the von Swithington family. I was not culturally and ethnocentrically in tune with them. Their progenitors were at the hunt club while mine were hawking *schmates* on Hester Street.

I was asked by Mrs. von Swithington: "Doctor, when can Algernon and I resume sexual congress?" I looked at my watch and said: "Four-thirty!" I got the blank look. I then recouped and gave the proper answer which, in this case, for the benefit of Algernon, I said: "In four years."

My lack of cultural and societal cognizance of the von Swithington family worked against me. It made humor inappropriate. I realized that the gap between us was unbridgeable when I overheard Mrs. von Swithington asking the waitress in our hospital coffee shop the proper name of those "circular Jewish breakfast rolls."

Are the Teitelbaums funnier than the von Swithingtons? No they are not. The von Swithingtons are hilarious *in their own societal and cultural context*. My interaction with both families had to be tailored. I was in tune with the former but not with the latter.

Humor is also an important defense mechanism for the physician. It is easy to be consumed by the seriousness of medicine. Humor is used to offset that seriousness.

Residents should not use humor with patients. Frankly, they have not earned the right to use it. They can use it sparingly in conferences and among attendings. Their use of humor should be reserved for the senior years of their residency.

A final word about humor.

Any witticism, *bon mot* or *mot juste* uttered by an attending physician is hilariously insightful and humorous. This is called the privilege of the attending. Residents who understand this get better recommendations and letters of reference.

As for chiefs of surgery - for the resident who wishes to succeed in his program - they are uniformly witty and downright hilarious.

Matrix Lesson 82

Do not create pathology in an
attempt to define pathology

A focal point for the discussion of any surgical complication is the extent of the procedure. The more extensive the procedure, the higher the incidence of complications. Was the procedure too limited? Did the procedure do more than it should have done?

Matrix Lesson #82 examines the situation in which the surgical team, in its quest to define surgical pathology, *creates* surgical pathology, thereby complicating the clinical situation.

This is best analyzed in the context of surgical technique. Good surgical technique is based on "tissue sense." Tissue sense is the surgical talent that lets a surgeon know what he can do to what tissue at what time under what circumstances.

I suppose it could be quantified by affixing a tensiometer to the hands of a gifted surgeon and chart out what could be done to which tissues under varying circumstances.

But it is more than that. Tissue sense is an appreciation for human tissue in all of its diverse states. Why will one surgeon wind up with three enterotomies during surgery for a bowel obstruction while another surgeon will have none? Why will the dissection be bloody in one case, yet not in a similar case performed by another surgeon? The answer has a lot to do with the surgeon's tissue sense. Tissue sense can be learned, but it is one of the hardest surgical talents to acquire. Thankfully, the evolution of the human body has provided us with the fibroblast and the macrophage: two cell types that can, to some degree, help the patient survive a surgeon with little tissue sense.

For example, a patient is being operated on for a small bowel obstruction. During a search for the obstructing mechanism, enterotomies are created in distended loops of bowel, complicating the procedure. The technical error of misjudging the fragility of the tissue led to this problem. New pathology (enterotomy with the morbidity arising from it) has been created, complicating the already existing pathology (the mechanism causing the small bowel obstruction). Matrix Lesson #82 has been learned.

"New pathology has been created in an attempt to define existing pathology which, in this case, was resolving."

By learning this valuable lesson, surgical residents will become more aware of their ability to create pathology and to complicate their lives and their patients' lives.

But Lesson #82 does not apply just to operative surgery.

A patient is recovering from a perforated ulcer. He is tolerating a regular diet. A low-grade fever and right upper quadrant pain develop. A chest film reveals a small right pleural effusion and leads the team to suspect a sub-hepatic collection. The following day the patient has no fever and is hungry. The CAT scan ordered the night before, however, proceeds, revealing a small collection in the right sub-hepatic area. The team proceeds to a needle catheter drainage. A large right hepatic hematoma develops which requires laparotomy. The patient is dismissed one week later. New pathology has been created in an attempt to define existing pathology which, in this case, was resolving.

There are unlimited opportunities to create pathology in today's medical center. It is one of the contradictory themes running through medicine that our attempt to stamp out disease through technologic sophistication has often created new diseases.

Do not create pathology in an attempt to detect pathology!

Matrix Lesson 83

Master the art of the postoperative
family meeting

One of the current core competencies of medical
education today is "professionalism." I cannot define this
word, other than to say it's what your parents should
have taught you in high school. Nowhere is
professionalism more on display than when meeting with
patients' families.

Talking to families is just as much a surgical talent as
learning to place the posterior row of sutures. It is a talent
that is seldom formally taught in surgical curricula.

The best way for residents to learn how to talk to
families is to accompany the attending surgeon into the
surgical waiting area. I learned how to talk to families by
standing beside the masters. I learned how not to talk to
families by standing beside several inarticulate surgeons.

The classroom for this lesson is the surgical waiting area. This area is a collection of chairs and tables outside of every operating theater. In a larger sense, it is the confluence of the extended families of surgical pathology. Behind every tumor, aneurysm, obstruction and gallstone is a patient and an extended patient family. These people must be addressed following the operation.

Everyone in the waiting area has two things in common. They have a relative or friend, who has undergone an operation. And, lurking in their minds is the fact that some day, at some time, they will be patients on the other side of the wall between the waiting area and the operating room.

Families want to hear only one thing after an operation. "She's fine" (particularly if the patient is female). Once that is stated, families remember little else, so it is important that the surgeon makes an effort to put the operation into some perspective for the family.

I divide family conversations into the answers of the five surgical questions:

■ How did the operation go?

In simple and straightforward language, describe the operation, particularly if it differed from pre-operative discussions. Explain why. This need not be lengthy or detailed. The time for length and detail is before surgery.

■ What was found and what was done?

Were there any changes from the pre-operative plans? Were there any unexpected findings? And if so, how might these changes influence the postoperative course?

■ What can be expected in the postoperative course?

Were there any findings that might lead to problems that were not discussed pre-operatively? What concerns do I, as the operating surgeon, have which the family should be aware of?

It is best to assume that the family knows nothing about the postoperative state. You may be worried about a subphrenic abscess or rebleed, while they are concerned about the nasogastric tube.

■ Where will the patient be and when can they be seen?

All families want to see their friends or relatives after surgery. They uniformly ask when they can be seen.

■ Will you be available?

Families are concerned about weekend and night coverage, vacations and other events that might cause the operating surgeon to be absent. It is helpful and allays anxiety to explain any absences which might arise.

"Talking to families is just as much a surgical talent as learning to place the posterior row of sutures. It is a talent that is seldom formally taught in surgical curricula."

The families of surgical patients are experiencing a once in a lifetime event. The surgeon is experiencing a two or three times a day event. The gap between the two experiences must be bridged by this postoperative discussion.

The family could not care less that you constructed an isoperistaltic antecolic gastrojejunostomy, that there was a pre-ductal portal vein or that you used Smedly-Jones' technique.

They want to hear, in simple terms, how things played out and what concerns the surgeon may have.

Hospitals that recognize the importance of the postoperative discussion usually have a family room or "quiet room" for these discussions or meeting. A cold and spare open area restricts surgical discussions and contributes to a general uneasiness.

Some of the most discomfiting waiting room experiences arise when the surgical technocrat takes over. When diagrams, intestinal loops, and vascular anastomoses dominate the discussion, compassion and understanding suffer.

Thankfully, some medical schools have recognized the need to develop communication skills in their students. Somewhere in the late 1970s medical schools recognized that even surgeons would have to relate to families. They began teaching courses in interpersonal skills. I think some of the professors who taught those courses have talk shows now in which people vent their feelings.

This facet of surgical life, unfortunately, is not taught at the resident level. Residents can learn how to talk to families by making waiting room visits with the attending surgeon an essential part of "the operation."

Matrix Lesson #83 stresses the importance of learning to talk to surgical families.

Matrix Lesson 84

When all else fails, order a physical exam

Since the introduction of the CAT scan, the importance of the time-honored "complete physical exam" has declined. Why would we listen for whispering pectoriloquy when we have a machine that can pick up a 0.5cm lung nodule? Why should we check for a Forthergill sign when we have a machine that can look deep within the soul of the rectus?

Matrix Lesson #84 does not address the initial physical examination. It reminds us that this medical ritual may need to be resurrected in the postoperative period.

The medical day can be a hurried and frenetic affair. Add several intensive care unit patients and one has the potential for missed physical findings on postoperative patients.

It is natural to get into a rounds routine in the postoperative period. If these rounds are going smoothly, one may let his guard down, particularly on busy days.

"A repeat (or initial) complete physical examination plays a vital role in the evaluation of postoperative complications."

Here's a list of findings on physical examination:

- Bilateral orchitis.

This patient weighed over three hundred pounds. He had undergone an open appendectomy and developed postoperative fever. Only when the imaging physician* pointed out two swollen scrotal spheres on the CT scan was the surgical teams' interest directed to the genitalia. Buried between these massive thighs were two red-hot swollen testicles.

- Peri-rectal abscess.

How can a patient develop a surgically significant peri-rectal abscess after a cholecystectomy? There are two possibilities: the patient had the abscess on admission and it was not detected on physical examination; or, the patient developed the abscess during the postoperative period and it was not considered as part of the differential of postoperative fever.

After the HIDA scan, the CAT scan and after the ERCP, a physical examination revealed the abscess.

- Cellulitis of the back caused by (I'm not kidding) a syringe plunger embedded in edematous tissue.

* The physician formerly known as the radiologist.

I will not regale the reader with the cryptic report: "Foreign body in left thorax."

▩ A colo-vaginal fistula.

Point made.

Each of the above diagnoses was made by physical exam on patients who developed postoperative problems. Each of these diagnoses was made after various investigative studies had been ordered and in most cases, performed. (My favorite is the chest X-ray showing the syringe plunger.)

A repeat (or initial) complete physical examination plays a vital role in the evaluation of postoperative complications. There is even more of a role for such an exam if the patient has had a lengthy stay.

Oddly, seeing a patient daily makes it tougher to pick up subtle findings, particularly if the patient is not that ill. There is a law of conservation of surgical energy which states that we save our energies for sick patients, not for patients with lingering or ill-defined problems. Sometimes conserving that energy causes us to limit our physical examinations. Surgeons tend to focus on the area of surgery. Our guard may be let down if we frequently see the patient.

To order the test known as a physical exam, one fills out a requisition and writes: "Complete physical exam on 704 Bed 1." The requisition is then forwarded to a physician who has never seen the patient before, for he is in the best position to conduct a general physical exam and detect such pathology as is listed above.

Lesson #84 takes on particular importance for the AM admission patient. There is usually an interval between the office visit and the operation. During that time new findings may have developed.

When all else fails, order a physical examination!

Matrix Lesson 85

Forget the CV

Discover the CV

Guest physicians are frequent visitors to the Matrix Conference. They usually appear when they are asked to give grand rounds. Attending this conference is usually part of their itinerary. The audience may have been supplied with a copy of the guest's CV (curriculum vitae).

The CV is a physician's single most descriptive document. It lists personal data and academic data. Matrix Lesson #85 teaches us to learn to differentiate between the traditional CV and the meaningful CV.

Let me explain.

The reader is familiar with the standard medical CV (curriculum vitae - literally, the pathway of the life). This is the usual list of birth-place, location, educational background and achievements. This list is usually recited before lectures or included with applications or depositions.

I have read and listened to hundreds of these lists. They are all presented in a familiar pattern. Everyone graduated. Everyone is boarded. Everyone has a list of publications.

What does one really learn about the individual from this type of CV? Not much!

> "We must revamp the form of the CV. We must redefine the meaning of the CV. We must get back to its original intent."

The curriculum vitae, as currently delivered, has the tone of reading a criminal his Miranda rights. In fact, the CV, in its current form, is a sort of academic Miranda pronouncement:

- You have the right to graduate from a prestigious medical school.
- You have the right to join local and national medical societies.
- You have the right to reach attending level at several hospitals.
- You have the right to write and publish several papers which will neither be read nor will ever benefit any human.
- You have the right to two diplomas. If you cannot afford a diploma one will be provided for you.

These elements of life are usually recited in a droning monotone. The standard CV has all of the makings of a boring and somewhat meaningless document.

We must revamp the form of the CV. We must redefine the meaning of the CV. We must get back to its original intent.

It will do us well to recapture some of the excitement of the original meaning of the word *curriculum*. The curriculum in ancient Rome was the path the Roman chariots took during their frantic races in the Coliseum. How is it that this exciting activity with such a rich history is now equated with the rote chanting of relatively common accomplishments? Why hasn't the fire and excitement of Charlton Heston beating his horse senseless crossed the millenia and presented itself at grand rounds introductions?

We need a new approach to the standard CV and that approach is called ... the CV!

The CV to which I am referring is the *curriculum veritae* - the true path and outline of a physician's life. This CV is not a droning litany of academic progression. It is a fiery statement of the central core of the individual. It is the true path of life. It is the essence of the individual.

The curriculum veritae tells an audience what type of person the physician is in real terms - human terms that all can appreciate. One has no idea of the person himself by saying that he "spent four years at the NIH studying plasma."

But one has a better idea if the introduction reads:

  ▧   Dr. Carlson has been divorced three times. Despite ridiculous settlements against him necessitating his working four jobs to keep up alimony payments, he continues to work closely with the resident staff; or

  ▧   Dr. Krassner was sued last year for delay in diagnosis of a breast cancer. Despite a sensational and much publicized trial, he continued to treat his patients and colleagues with the respect and devotion for which he is noted; or

  ▧   Dr. Milburn is a fly-fisherman whose surgical income supports his hobby; or

■   despite a declining case load, a practice decimated by managed care and rapacious senior partners, Dr. Voss has maintained an upbeat character making it a pleasure to sit with him in the surgeons' lounge.

These are statements that give us insight into the true person. These are statements that evoke the excitement of the ancient chariot races. They get the blood pumping and the heart racing. They animate the core of the person's humanity.

These are statements that describe the person's true path through life - his curriculum veritae.

Matrix Lesson #85 teaches us to redefine the standard CV in an effort to examine the true path the physician has followed.

Matrix Lesson 86

Double-headers are for ballgames

During a presentation of a surgical complication, it may be revealed that two procedures were performed. A complication may have developed from the performance of the second procedure - a procedure that was not originally planned at the outset of the operation.

Consider these statements:

- Case #1. "The gallbladder was on a mesentery and since we were there ..."
- Case #2. "The appendix was in the field, and was readily accessible ..."
- Case #3. "The operation had gone well, and since the Meckel's diverticulum was clearly visible through this incision, we ..."

So begins the presentation of the complication.

We tempt the surgical gods with our desire to remove what is accessible and what *may* cause disease. We may embark on additional procedures when the primary procedure is completed.

I am not a medical nihilist. I appreciate the one lecture in epidemiology I received in medical school which stated the incidence and occurrence of disease. But I also realize that *each surgical procedure must be viewed as an independent procedure with its own set of risks and complications.*

"We tempt the surgical gods with our desire to remove what is accessible and what may cause disease."

Case #1 is a cholecystectomy with all of the risks of bleeding, ductal injury, bile leak and pancreatitis. Case #2 is an appendectomy with all of the risks of infection, small bowel obstruction and cecal fistulization. Case #3 is removal of a Meckel's with all of the risks of bleeding and anastomotic healing.

"Doc, as long as you're there can you take out my gallbladder?"

Thus begins the epic surgical folk-tale. How can a patient come to a surgeon with a relatively straightforward problem and how can that problem be compounded by the complications of an "ancillary" procedure?

There are solid indications to perform two operations at the same sitting. The most cogent one is the discovery of previously undetected pathology that represents an immediate threat to the patient: the hydrops of the gallbladder; the nearly obstructing colon lesion; the small bowel tumor; the pelvic mass in a female. These findings represent fairly solid indications for performing secondary procedures. But, as a general rule, double-headers are for Fenway Park and Wrigley Field.

Consider the risk of surgical complications for any ancillary or subordinate procedure. Weigh that risk against the benefit to the patient.

Matrix Lesson 87

Collect, read, study and master every surgical clinico-pathologic case published in the *New England Journal of Medicine*

New England has made many contributions to medicine. New England has given us Ted Williams, Larry Bird, Derek Sanderson and Tom Brady. New England has given us brown bread, Scollay Square and James Michael Curley. New England has also given us the *New England Journal of Medicine*.

New York may have invented the elements of a classical surgical education, but New England refined those elements into an educational whole and has presented them weekly since 1812.

Along with a general decline in the verbal skills of surgical house officers has arisen a lack of appreciation for this weekly element of classical surgical education.

In many traditional hospitals the weekly clinico-pathologic conference (CPC) was an essential part of the surgical educational process. During this conference, an invited guest was asked to give a differential diagnosis of a case that had been admitted to the hospital. Supposedly, the discussant did not know the diagnosis. He was expected to discuss the diagnostic possibilities.

"The clinico-pathologic conference, over and above any medical skills, also honed the skills of presentation, lucid thinking and deductive reasoning."

During my own surgical residency in the 1970s, a debate began as to the efficacy of these conferences as a teaching tool. This was just at the beginning of the technologic explosion of endoscopy, CAT scanning and interventional radiology. Some educators felt that the CPC was just theater and entertainment. They maintained that in this day (the then modern day of 1973) the CPC was an anachronism.

Others felt that the exercise was a valuable teaching tool, especially for residents unschooled in the discipline of rigorous case presentation. The latter group was correct.

The clinico-pathologic conference, over and above any medical skills, also honed the skills of presentation, lucid thinking and deductive reasoning. Its very structure fosters ongoing assessment of clinical skills. A physician is presented a problem. The radiologist has his say. The physician attempts a diagnosis. The correct diagnosis is revealed. Then the pathologist reviews the case, usually with a comment on the varying presentations. The CPC was a valuable exercise.

Fortunately, the *New England Journal of Medicine* has continued to publish CPCs. Their web access now allows downloading of photographs, radiographic images and charts. In 1973, some long-forgotten senior resident, observing my own pitiful verbal, organizational and intellectual skills, recommended that I read these weekly clinico-pathologic conferences with a special eye on CPCs of interest to a surgeon.

As with so many great strides in surgical education, this brilliant recommendation came from a work-a-day-type surgeon intent on improving his own diagnostic and surgical skills. Since that recommendation in 1973, I have collected the surgical CPCs from the *New England Journal of Medicine*.

Noting the contributions of David Letterman to American surgery, I assemble a Top Ten Surgical CPC list which I occasionally distribute to the resident staff *. How does a CPC make my Top Ten list? I have four criteria:

   The quality of the discussion by the discussant.

I do not care if his final diagnosis is correct. What I do care about is the skill, specificity, style and interest level he maintains during his discussion. Droning, pontificating, and surgical arcana may lead to tenure, but it will not lead to my ten best surgical CPC list!

   The quality of the bibliography.

The CPC bibliographies are a readily available reference for me in researching all kinds of surgical problems. They are current. They are usually excellent papers. Even better, they portray current treatment as a historical progression, listing the landmark papers for the disease state.

   The level of the discussion presented by the pathologist or radiologist.

* If you are interested in my recent Top Ten Surgical CPC list send me an e-mail at MatrixPearls@Gmail.com.

The role of the pathologist and radiologist has declined in many conference settings. Many surgical educators feel that an active role by the pathologist and radiologist is essential to any surgical conference. Their active participation at Matrix Conferences, interdisciplinary conferences, and grand rounds makes these meetings more interesting and generally elevates the level of discussion. They represent the entry point (radiology) and exit point (pathology) for all disease. They define disease, expand on the implications of the surgical findings and often enhance the case by tying together various elements of the clinical presentation of the disease.

▪ The response to questions at the end of the discussion.

Even though nuance and voice inflection cannot be detected from a written text, in the selections I have made they do come through and often answer questions the reader may have posed.

Matrix Lesson #87 mandates the collection and mastery of the *New England Journal of Medicine* surgical CPCs.

What does the CPC teach?

▪ The CPC teaches the resident how to develop a differential diagnosis.
▪ The CPC teaches the resident the proper method of presenting that diagnosis in the context of the case at hand.
▪ The CPC gives the resident diagnostic models for common presenting symptoms.
▪ The CPC teaches the resident the value of collecting CPCs for his own case presentations.

Matrix Lesson #87 resurrects the CPC as a valuable teaching tool for all residents.

Lesson #87 will turn that disheveled sleep-deprived collection of residents into literate, conversant and medically sophisticated practitioners.

Matrix Lesson 88

Learn the art of sitting

When I am on my deathbed at a major teaching hospital, thoughts of resident surgical life will pass through my addled mind.

In the gray dawn of early morning rounds, several white-cloaked people will stand and mumble at my bedside. It is as if a ritual religious service is about to begin in a medieval monastery. In this ritual, the acolytes must, before the prayers begin, assemble in a semicircular manner established by their rank. They must stand at the bedside before beginning their work. They bring out their prayer books and mumble, only to leave as I emerge from the arms of Morpheus.

As I emerge, I wonder: "What happened at my bedside? Was it a dream? Was it real or was it some drug-induced apparition? I know I have doctors, but these ghostly visitors could not be from my world." They appear. They stand. They mumble. They disappear into the mists of the morning. Such is the custom of rounding in teaching hospitals.

"Sitting is a powerful body signal. It tells the patient that you have the time to focus on his problem."

Unlike the dawn visitors, some surgeons have the unique ability to make every patient feel that as if they are the only patient on the service. I had partners like that. Despite multiple emergencies, difficult cases and the exigencies of the surgical day, these physicians could make anyone feel as if his problem, no matter how small or insignificant, is the only problem in the hospital at that time. What a wonderful attribute for a physician!

Part of communicating that essential feeling is their simple habit of sitting down during their rounds. Sitting is a powerful body signal. It tells the patient that you have the time to focus on his problem.

I hate to sit down. It is time-consuming. Once you sit down you actually have to listen to all sorts of things - complaints, concerns, interests and apprehensions - the four horsemen of the inefficient surgical day.

My friend, mentor and confidante, Dr. Leon Morgenstern, reviewing his own illustrious surgical teaching career, wrote: "During many years of practice, I had witnessed countless flying visits by both house staff and attending physicians, alone or in concert. Standing by the edge of the bed or towering over the patient at bedside, encounters were short, polite and often perfunctory. The importance of the visit was eclipsed by the pressures of time and tasks undone. Yet, for the patient this was the event of the day - the doctor's visit is unmatched in importance by anything else that occurs before or after."*

Dr. Morgenstern is right. His eloquent plea to sit down during rounds is the foundation for Matrix Lesson #88. Even if just the most junior member of the team sits down, the meaning is conveyed. It is my hope that this lesson will be learned in the context of the newly implemented eighty-hour work week.

There is now time for this most basic of surgical actions.

Morgenstern L. The Art of Sitting. *West J Med* 1994; 161: 93.

Matrix Lesson 89

Learn diagnostic restraint

"Corollary of Law #89: do not chase rainbows."

The patient suffered a perforated diverticulitis ten days ago. The colostomy is functioning well. The patient looks great. He is enjoying his regular diet. The temperature, however, is 100.2. Because of this temperature elevation, the infectious disease consultant wants a CAT scan.

This study will prove that the retroperitoneum is distorted and edematous. It may show some fluid. It may show some thickening.

In short, this study will show what is already known - anatomic distortion results from pathology and surgery.

That distortion, in a stable and improving patient, is usually not surgically significant. These findings, however, will undoubtedly fan the flames of internal medical angst. They will create what I call the *yentification** of an easily explained finding. They will saddle the managing surgeon and his patient with doubts and concerns which, in the face of clinical improvement, are needless.

What about the fluid? What about the thickening? In their attempt to define that which is already known they may create a diagnostic worry-swirl that does no-one - especially the patient - any good.

A rainbow has been chased. Regrettably, no pot of gold has been found. Gravity has been rediscovered (postoperative changes seen on CAT scan).

The popular HIDA scan, often falsely positive in a variety of general surgical conditions, is also a common rainbow-chasing ploy.

There are many causes for right upper quadrant pain in the postoperative surgical patient. It is well, however, to keep in mind that the HIDA scan may be falsely positive in such states. Many a Matrix Conference has begun with: "We wish to present an error in diagnosis - a normal gallbladder removed with a pre-operative diagnosis of postoperative acalculous cholecystitis, suggested by a positive HIDA scan."

Save the investigative studies for a time when there is a medically probable chance of finding pathology!

Don't chase rainbows. Consider the lesson of exercising diagnostic restraint.

---

*Yentification - transformation of lucid medical thought into fuzzy technobabble, unlikely to result in patient benefit.

Matrix Lesson 90

Never say: "Never let the sun rise nor
set on a small bowel obstruction"

Complications of surgery for small bowel obstruction are frequently listed on the weekly complications list. When the complication arises from a delay in diagnosis, someone will state: "Never let the sun rise nor set on a small bowel obstruction."

This statement is deeply ingrained into the surgical soul. Passed on from generation to generation as a grand oral tradition, this statement has been repeated and has been codified into a conference litany.

As a resident, I was taught that this statement was categorically true. As a clinical surgeon, I can say that frequently it is not. Many thousands of patients have been subjected to needless explorations as a knee-jerk surgical reaction to this statement.

I suppose, at one time, during the early days of laparotomy, there was some reasonable foundation for this mantra. It cautioned surgeons to avoid neglecting the patient with the bowel obstruction. It meant that it is often difficult to separate complete bowel obstruction from incomplete bowel obstructions. It meant that one cannot reliably differentiate strangulating obstruction from non-strangulating obstruction. But it does not mean that every patient with an air-fluid level requires surgery! Nor does it mean that every patient with a radiology report which reads "consistent with small bowel obstruction" needs surgery.

"Never let the sun rise nor set on a patient with a small bowel obstruction who, after careful evaluation in the studied judgment of the responsible surgeon, will not improve."

It does not mean that judicious re-evaluation of the patient after hydration, assessment and decompression should be subordinated to some narrow professorial law formulated in the late 1930s.

Who uttered this for the first time? Was it William Osler? Was it Sir Zachary Cope? Was it Zachary Taylor? Was it Elizabeth Taylor? I do not know. But this statement has been passed down to every surgical intern who ever went to an emergency room. It has restricted the judicious analysis of the patient who may have a small bowel obstruction.

One of the revelations of my surgical career was the first time I witnessed the violation of this old saw. My partner was called to the emergency room to see a patient with a small bowel obstruction. Many years earlier, the patient had been operated upon for a perforated appendix. The film was consistent with a small bowel obstruction. The patient was afebrile, mildly dehydrated, had a softly distended abdomen and a normal white count. The patient was comfortable. Yet there was the film. The report read "small bowel obstruction."

I called surgery. My partner inserted a nasogastric tube and canceled the call to surgery. He suggested we re-evaluate the patient later on in the day. The patient improved. Two days later he was dismissed from the hospital.

My partner had violated a professorial edict. My partner demonstrated a more sophisticated knowledge of bowel obstruction than I had. He treated a patient, not a film.

Let me enhance this old saw and properly phrase it as Matrix Lesson #90: never let the sun rise nor set on a patient with a small bowel obstruction who, after careful evaluation in the studied judgment of the responsible surgeon, will not improve.

Revamping this old saw is long overdue. Besides, what about the surgeons in Lapland?

Matrix Lesson 91

The last doctor is always the smartest doctor

As a surgical consultant I have frequently observed residents who are called upon to evaluate patients. Many times these patients will be at the end of their evaluations at a point in time when the need for surgery is clear.

The resident arrives, reviews the lab data and the workup. The resident then gives the surgical benediction - "yes, surgery is needed."

This makes the resident feel good. It re-enforces what he already knows. There is a tendency in such situations to overestimate the amount of knowledge needed to give this benediction. While there is always a role for refined surgical judgment and suggestions for further studies, many times the surgeon will decide to do what has already been decided to do. This does not take a large amount of (dare I use the word) "cognition."

I am not a fan of the eight-day laborious medical service workup for common diseases. I am not a fan of Occam's Razor violations (see Matrix Lesson #36).

But I do recognize that as a consultant, I am often the beneficiary of other physicians' hard work. Surgeons often see the patient with the pathology already delineated and the plan for surgery as part of the differential approach. We are summoned to verify what is generally already known.

> "But I do recognize that as a consultant, I am often the beneficiary of other physicians' hard work."

In these situations, we are the "last doctor" on the case. By virtue of work already completed, we are the "smartest." We know everything because it has been laid out for us. Based on that work, we plan our operation. Being the last doctor is fun. Being the "smartest" doctor is even more fun. But our role in these cases must be put into perspective lest we overestimate our skills and become afflicted with that debilitating surgical disease - hubris (see Matrix Lesson #75).

Matrix
Lesson 92

Consider the *shtick** that accompanies the test

The Matrix Conference frequently analyzes complications arising from investigative studies. It is important to remember that every test ordered has a *shtick* associated with it.

If a CAT scan is ordered, the nurse immediately brings in an oil drum full of water-soluble contrast (the hospital equivalent to the minimart "supertanker," "big gulp" or "super big gulp").

The nurse dutifully puts a straw in this hypertonic slurry and says to the patient: "Drink it!" This is a lot like those beer-chugging contests that were so popular in the 1960s. The problem is that instead of a nineteen-year-old

---

* *Shtick* - a Yiddish word meaning the stuff surrounding a thing or a person. The identifying characteristics of a thing. The shtick is the smaller details that are part of a greater something.

linebacker, the recipient of the "contrast challenge" is usually a debilitated octogenarian with an ileus and an impaired swallowing mechanism. The shtick associated with the study may do the patient in. Consider it.

A pelvic ultrasound may be accompanied by efforts to fill the bladder to better delineate the pelvic anatomy. This involves the infusion of intravenous fluid to distend the bladder. The next time you have trouble sitting through a double feature sipping the "mug-o-cola," think about this requirement of pelvic sonography.

"There is a shtick surrounding
every diagnostic study!
Know the shtick!"

And finally, the colon studies of which we are so fond. There is an oral cathartic whose instructions are basically: place seven liters of this at the bedside and instruct the patient to drink it over two hours. This fluid, packaged in styrofoam peanuts, transported only at night over little used country roads, is a volatile, chemically unstable tenia splitter. It is hygroscopic. This medicine could easily dehydrate the famous "well nourished 72kg male" we all read about in medical school. Consider this shtick when it is placed at the bedside of an elderly patient whose daily liquid intake is three cups of tea and three croutons.

There is a shtick surrounding every diagnostic study! Know the shtick!

I formulated and codified Lesson #92 after my own personal experience with a diagnostic study centered on the colon.

Matrix Lesson 93

Beware the "senior surgeon"

The better Matrix Conferences are the polite Matrix Conferences. Residents are not referred to by their first name. Chiefs are given great deference. Older surgeons are also given that same deference by virtue of their age or long service to the hospital. They may be referred to as "senior surgeons."

The origin of the term "senior surgeon" is obscure. There is no such designation within any governing body of surgery. No organization has ever defined it. I have never seen a formal hospital staff bylaw definition.

I have always found it quite interesting that the person who first applies this term is usually the surgeon himself during a discussion with a patient or with a junior colleague.

This mysterious category of senior surgeon probably originated from surgeons who were approaching retirement. They noticed a decreasing caseload, an avalanche of new surgical methods and an increasingly competitive environment. To combat the ravages of a senescent practice, they most likely began describing themselves with this term as a means of impressing patients. They engaged in surgical hagiography - the rewriting of their own surgical history with the goal of glorification.

This is totally understandable. Surgery is an intensely personal discipline. Combine this with the fact that we often forget our failures and revel in our successes, and one can see the penchant for self-enhancement.

In many conferences, however, the term "senior surgeon" gives rise to a few knowing smirks. "Senior surgeon" for some is a euphemism for old surgeons, past their prime, who came through in a day when there was credit for past performance.

"This mysterious category of 'senior surgeon' probably originated from surgeons who were approaching retirement."

In the embattled calling that is general surgery today, there is no credit for past performance. Getting a current, knowledgeable opinion from a senior surgeon is difficult, since many are backward looking instead of forward looking. This is not an indictment of outdated surgical thought as much as it is a fact of advancing age.

Senior surgeons frequently attend the Matrix Conference. A moderator who does not understand the essence of "senior surgeons" may call on them for comments. He does not realize that when these men trained, a haruspex* was an integral member of the surgical team.

* The haruspex was the person in ancient Rome who would inspect the entrails of a sacrificial victim in order to divine the future.

When they speak, there may be a mish-mash of myth, outdated practice, folklore and the sweet reverie of days gone by. If there were boards in nostalgia, many senior surgeons would be the examiners.

Senior surgeons do, however, fill a larger surgical need. Most of them carry themselves well. They *look* like they know something. They fulfill the television viewers' ideal of the concerned doctor, riding through the snow in Vermont.

They are excellent surgical ambassadors for the public relations aspects of general surgery. In addition, they engender respect for age - combating an increasingly frequent cultural deficiency. They also have a healthy respect and interest in surgical history.

For these reasons their presence at the Matrix Conference is valuable.

It will be divine justice, having recorded the above for posterity if, in the not too distant future, I am found doddering around a medical center in plaid urine-stained bell-bottoms, telling an orderly that "I'm a senior surgeon!"

Two young surgical residents will look at each other, and will say: "What can happen to a person!"

Matrix Lesson 94

When common sense interferes with
a protocol, follow common sense

- "Dr. Warren always takes down the splenic flexure this way."
- "Dr. Smithers always works up a suspected pulmonary embolus with these tests."
- "The decision tree for the fixed pancreatic head mass says we should ..."
- "Here is the algorithm for the obstructing ascending colon lesion."
- "The radiologic protocol for a barium enema is to get spot films of each flexure."

Medicine, particularly surgery, is full of protocols. Protocols are handy frameworks for dealing with common diseases. They can often simplify problems by building on past approaches to those problems. They are helpful for the junior residents who may not have seen the problem before. Fortunately, most disease states fall into predictable patterns which allow standard approaches to their diagnosis and treatment. Those standard approaches become surgical protocol. Nevertheless, a protocol or algorithm may sometimes contradict the most powerful force in clinical surgery - the physician's common sense.

Laparoscopic extraction of common bile duct stones is a good example. This innovative technique, an offshoot of laparoscopic cholecystectomy, offers the patient with common duct stones nearly the same recovery as the laparoscopic cholecystectomy patient. There may be a fixed protocol for retrieving such stones. It may include the passage of wires and baskets followed by choledochoscopy. Sometimes the protocol can be tedious, time-consuming and, at a certain point, futile.

At that point, a common sense judgment is made by the surgeon and other approaches to the bile duct stones are used. Common sense has interfered with a protocol.

Radiologists may not recognize the common-sense/protocol border during semi-urgent contrast studies for colon lesions. Their protocol may say to get spot films of each flexure and examine the cecum. If a nearly obstructing descending colon lesion is seen, common sense says to stop there, lest the cecum be filled with hypertonic fluid, distend and create a bigger problem than originally faced. Common sense here says to terminate the study and terminate the protocol.

"Nevertheless, a protocol or algorithm may sometimes contradict the most powerful force in clinical surgery - the physician's common sense."

The use of oral contrast is part of the protocol for some other investigative studies, yet common sense may say the patient should not drink fluids. A cursory look into a patient's room often proves the point. You are hurrying to the office and glance at your patient with a resolving bowel obstruction. Some member of the team has ordered a CAT scan. The picture is indelibly printed in your mind as you see a vat of contrast with a straw in it being forced upon your patient. The protocol says drink it; common sense says do not drink it.

It is as well to look at the history of the word *protocol* to try to link it to common sense. Protocol comes from the Latin *protocollum*, which was the first leaf or page of a volume. If I were writing such an inscription on the first page of a textbook of clinical surgery, I would have Matrix Lesson #94 as the protocollum.

Matrix Lesson 95

They can always hit you harder

The heyday of Lesson #95 passed with the inception of the eighty-hour work-week. I include this lesson for the attending surgeons, unencumbered by the need to develop a life-style and a need to pay attention to their psychosocial and ethno-cultural development.

After a string of surgical emergencies comes a natural tendency for working surgeons to feel that things will quiet down for a few hours. There is a belief that if one works very hard for a set period of time that certain dues would have been paid and a "light" period will follow. That respite will allow you to rest and ready yourself for the next onslaught. This makes cosmological sense; it makes no surgical sense.

You have worked up the four admissions for tomorrow, scrubbed on the trauma case, placed a central line on the medical service, prepared the seminar on tertiary pseudohyperaldosteronism, counseled the new intern and reported to the chief resident.

It is now 3:45AM. Prevailing wisdom dictates that there will be a break in the action, but ... the ER calls, the bleeder re-bleeds and the intern forgot what you said ...

> "There is a belief that if one works very hard for a set period of time that ... a 'light' period will follow ... This makes cosmological sense; it makes no surgical sense."

Matrix Lesson #95 crystallized during the famous blizzard of '78 in Boston. We had been up the night before with many emergencies. We were ready for a break. We knew that break would be upon us because of the arrival of a blizzard. We were convinced that we would have a slow and quiet night because the blizzard was supposed to be the largest winter storm in fifty years. The snow began. The blizzard worsened. The city shut down.

No staff or resident could leave the hospital. Nothing was moving. No patients could leave. No patients could arrive. The expressways, even the famous "central artery" (which I always thought was a marvelous name for a freeway in a city so rich in medical history) was closed. We were exhausted. We could relax. Trapped in the hospital, our minds turned to other less medically oriented activities. The respite we deserved was upon us.

My beeper went off to call the emergency room. How could this be? No-one could possibly get to the emergency room. In the emergency room, I was confronted by four sleet-encrusted Massachusetts National Guardsmen carrying a stretcher. On that stretcher lay an 83-year-old female nursing home patient with an incarcerated femoral hernia.

The seed of Matrix Lesson #95 was firmly planted. They can always hit you harder!

Matrix Lesson 96

Never be afraid to cry uncle

"Corollary of Law #96: remember Libby Zion."

No resident on my current service reacts when I go up to them and ask: "Who is Libby Zion?"* Yet, every resident in America should know her name and the issues raised by her death.

I will not review the Zion case, nor will I make any judgments about it. I will only say that there is a middle

Laine C, Goldman L, Soukup JR, Hayes JG. The Impact of a Regulation Restricting Medical House Staff Working Hours on the Quality of Patient Health Care. JAMA 1993; 269: 374-8.
See also Farber MA. "Who Killed Libby Zion?" Vanity Fair, December 1988: 190.
See also "Jury Divides Blame in Hospital Death." New York Times, February 7, 1995: A11.

ground between the Draconian "I did it so you have to do it" approach to surgical training and the "get in touch with your feelings" school of resident education.

The disparity between these two approaches to medical education was a central theme of the Zion trial and the subsequent legislation that arose from this trial.

It is impractical to run a surgical residency on an eight to five basis. It is essential that surgical residents weather a storm. To some degree, surgical training should mirror the entity it was designed to master - surgical pathology. Surgical pathology is ruthless, neverending, sneaky and totally unforgiving. It is the most formidable enemy known to man and to woman.

"If a resident or a staff surgeon is sleep-deprived and cannot function, he or she should cry 'uncle' and get relief."

As one masters the craft of surgery, there is a tendency to believe that along with that mastery comes an immunity from the effects of fatigue. You are the surgeon. You can't get tired. This is a byproduct of the "total immersion" approach to surgical education. It is very effective, but has never taken into account the injurious effects of fatigue.

Anything less than a total immersion surgical education program produces surgeon manqués, not surgeons. I participated in such a total immersion program. A perusal of my call schedule showed sixty-hour stretches and every-other-night stints.

Unfortunately, such a demanding approach leads to sleep deprivation. Sleep deprivation leads to corner-cutting and corner-cutting may lead to errors. Some of these errors may be fatal. As Vince Lombardi said: "Fatigue makes a coward of us all." It causes us to compromise.

If a resident or a staff surgeon is sleep-deprived and cannot function, he or she should cry "uncle" and get relief.

This approach calls for a delicate balance between the famous surgical macho image and the practicalities of bare-bones survival. Surgical educators must wrestle with this problem and should design schedules that allow for residents who are beyond fatigue to get relief.

There should be a mechanism in every call schedule (resident and staff) for rested, reliable and understanding back-up for those times when the winds of surgical fate have blown too much work your way.

A surgical education program and a surgical practice are demanding entities. Each of us remembers instances when the demands of residency or practice simply outstripped our ability to meet them.

When that point is reached, remember Matrix Lesson #96. Cry uncle and get some help.

Matrix Lesson 97

Be familiar with the civil justice system

There is a parallel universe running alongside the world of clinical medicine. That universe is the civil justice system. Currently, the civil justice system is the microscope through which our profession is being examined.

As you are reading this page, a surgeon is being cross-examined in a courtroom; another surgeon is conferring with his defense attorney; another surgeon is performing an expert review of a surgical case; and a jury is trying to figure out just what the hell is a duodenum!

No surgeon has ever been sued for a case that went well. We are only sued for cases that did not go well and that resulted in a death or a complication.

It is the task of the civil justice system to sort out these cases, decide which case has merit and to adjudicate the case.

It is not hyperbole to state that every surgical complication will be reviewed, at some point, by an attorney. For that reason, every member of the surgical team should be familiar with the principles of medical liability.

"Surgeons should understand the anatomy of a lawsuit ... the deposition process, the settlement process and even the trial process."

Surgeons should know the legal definitions of "standard of care," "reasonable medical probability," "proximate cause" and "assumption of the risk." Surgeons should know the legal requirements for "informed consent." They should understand the elements of a medical negligence case.

What does the opposing attorney have to prove? What is the standard for that proof? Can the opposing attorney show that because of the surgeon's actions, the patient suffered injury? Did that injury arise from the surgeon's actions or did those injuries arise from the disease itself?

Surgeons should understand the anatomy of a lawsuit. They should understand the deposition process, the settlement process and even the trial process. Failing to understand this process fails to recognize this parallel universe.

The job of the Matrix Conference is to analyze a complication, not to set a standard of care. Although many cases discussed may go on to litigation, the rules of Matrix discussions are quite different than the rules of civil justice.

The Matrix seeks perfection in surgical practice - an unattainable goal. Ideally, this search for perfection should set a constant goal of self-improvement and ongoing education. It is up to our legal brethren to explain to the public the difference between perfection and practice.

Matrix Lesson 98

Beware the AM admit!

When I came through my surgical education program, there was an entity called "the day before surgery admission." I know this may seem odd to younger readers, but patients were actually admitted to the hospital on the afternoon before their surgery.

Once admitted, their laboratory data would be assembled and collated. The anesthesiologist would visit them. The attending surgeon who would perform the procedure the next morning usually visited them.

Following these visits, the intern or resident would appear. The resident would take a history and examine the patient. A note would follow.

The patient went to sleep confident that the team had been assembled, the team had been briefed and everyone was on the same page.

"The AM admit is financial brilliance. The AM admit is educational stupidity."

Not a lot of medicine was practiced on this day before admission, but a lot was learned by the resident.

This admitting process was a central part of surgical education and practice. See the patient. Review the history. Examine the patient. Then correlate this interview and examination with the operative findings of the following morning.

This day before surgery admission was the perfect synthesis of observation, examination and correlation. To a large degree it was the heart of many surgical programs.

Then Bernie showed up!

Bernie was the accountant who sat down and suggested to the insurance companies that this "day before surgery" admission was a waste of money.

"Why," Bernie pleaded, "Should we pay for this extra day? It's costing us millions! Let's dump all of the responsibility of retrieving lab data, making sure there have been no changes in the patient's condition and other medical stuff onto the shoulders of the surgeon and the hospital! This will eliminate the need for admission the day prior to surgery!"

Bernie was a financial genius.

This explains why well-meaning patients who have paid their insurance premiums now must wake up at 4AM in the gray dawn of winter and schlep to a crowded pre-op cubicle just hours before an event that is arguably the most important event in their life.

It explains why these well-meaning people are thrust into the pre-operative chaos that is the pre-operative holding area of most hospitals.

Bernie explains the lost EKG. Bernie explains why the pre-operative history and physical examination is missing. Bernie explains why the lab data was faxed to the TGI Friday's in Haverhill rather than to the hospital. Bernie explains why cases are canceled, why surgeons are angry, why anesthesiologists are tearing their hair out and why nurses are frustrated. Bernie also explains why some of these AM admit patients wind up on the Matrix Conference complication list.

The AM admit is financial brilliance. The AM admit is educational stupidity. Bernie explains why the AM admit is a trap for the unwary surgeon. The process has added a huge burden to surgical practice.

Matrix Lesson #98 sensitizes us to the pitfalls of the AM admit process.

Matrix Lesson 99

Master the three As of a successful medical practice

When I went into practice, everyone knew what the "three As" of a successful practice were. This old saw had been around for a long time. It was perfectly logical to know them and understand them.

Every new attending realized the three As of success: availability, affability and ability. Be available and your practice will grow. Be affable and people will love to refer patients to you. If you are actually able to perform operations, that's even better.

You can't miss with the three As of medical practice. Since I only possessed two of these three As, I was never really wildly successful, but that's for another book.

Just as Matrix Lessons have redefined the meaning of the CV (Matrix Lesson #85) and the term C.E.O. (Matrix

Lesson #49), so has the surgical educational process changed the meaning of the three As of a successful practice.

The currently applicable three As have nothing to do with the personal qualities listed above. They deal with patient communication in an age of consumer awareness:

■   A#1. Alternatives.

It is the obligation of the surgeon to generally discuss alternative treatments with the patient. If appropriate, the patient has the right to know that non-surgical or different surgical treatments are available.

■   A#2. Additional opinions.

The term "second opinion" is well known to most patients. As the patient has become a "client," additional opinions have become part of the process of deciding to undergo surgery. In non-urgent difficult surgical situations, most surgeons welcome such opinions.

■   A#3. Available options.

The consultant surgeon should discuss care options with the patient. There are many ways to treat disease. A surgeon must consider the patient's age, risk factors, desires and expectations. Surgeons synthesize these elements into a surgical recommendation. If surgery is not an option, other options are discussed.

"The currently applicable three As have nothing to do with the personal qualities listed above. They deal with patient communication in an age of consumer awareness."

Progressing from the three As of early practice to the three As of Matrix Lesson #99 is part of professional maturation. Surgical experience, professional development and the realization that in the current practice of surgery there are many ways to treat diseases, led to the formulation of this lesson.

Matrix Lesson 100

Never ask the following questions:

"Would you drain it?"

"Should you drain it?"

"Did you drain it?"

There is a moment at every Matrix Conference when a specific question is asked. If that question is one of the three listed above *the discussion must end*.

General surgery - the queen of the medical specialties; the most demanding discipline on earth; the highest calling of humankind - has a morbid and debilitating latex fetish.

Quite simply, we are hung up on a piece of rubber. We discuss it at surgery. We opine on its benefits and management on rounds. We whittle it, suture it, place it and fashion it. We attach wall suction, hoping for a sump. We apply bulb suction, hoping for a seal. We are part of a silastic *opera bouffé*.

If one were to restrict his opinion of general surgeons to conversations in the surgeons' lounge or to the final comments at a Matrix Conference, one would have the overwhelming impression that the heart and sole of surgery is a six-inch piece of rubber.

One would think that at the national meetings, the keynote speaker would be the President of the Goodyear company. One would think that the anthem of the American Association of Surgeons would be the line from the song "High Hopes" that goes "Whoops, there goes another rubber tree plant." A rubber duckie logo would be emblazoned on various surgical diplomas and certificates. Sam Winston would be the chief of surgery. Drains. Drains. Drains. If general surgery needs a patron saint, it should be the Roman god, Vulcan.

In addition to the theoretical questions listed above, a second line of drain-oriented questioning invariably follows: "Did you use a J-P, a red rubber, a Chaffin-Pratt or a Pratt and Whitney?" "Was it a cigarette drain (regular or menthol?)?" "Did it sump?" "Was it open drainage or was it closed drainage?" (At this point the discussion sounds like an agricultural seminar.)

Following these discussions there is some mystical ranting about bacteria "swimming upstream." (This is the salmon-hatching theory of bacterial infection.)

A diatribe then ensues on drain removal. The third day? The fifth day? The seventh day? Was it "tweaked?" Was it advanced? Was it "cracked?"

A quasi-religious discussion centering on an inanimate object ensues. It is not a discussion of physiology, diagnostic expertise or pathology. It is not a discussion of practical surgical technique. It is an endless discussion about rubber.

Say what you will about the internists. They never discuss drains. That is their saving grace. Why are we discussing this issue? Why, deep in the surgical soul, is there an overwhelming need to discuss rubber? Why is the concept of drainage so indelibly imprinted on the surgical mind? Why after one hundred years of laparotomy, the development of powerful antibiotics and the imaging machines that can find pre-disease, are we still fixated on that pliable entity which the nurse routinely dips in water?

"We have been discussing its use on a weekly basis for over one hundred years. It is time to end the discussion."

To understand this mania we must remember the great contribution of Dr. Charles Bingham Penrose.* We must pay dutiful homage to this man, known in Vienna as Der Drainmeister.

Dr. Penrose sought a way around the adhesions formed by the simple gauze drains in use, at the time he was practicing. According to Abramson (vide infra), Dr. Penrose described his new drainage idea in his classic text A Textbook of Diseases of Women in 1897. He wrote: "To avoid this difficulty, the writer had for some time employed a drain made by surrounding the gauze bag with an ordinary rubber condom, the end of which has been cut open."

The Penrose drain was born.

We have been discussing its use on a weekly basis for over one hundred years. It is time to end the discussion.

Matrix Lesson #100 assures that questions regarding drainage will serve as the international sign to stop the discussion.

* For an entertaining vignette of this remarkable man, see Daniel J. Abramson. Charles Bingham Penrose and the Penrose Drain. SG&O 1976; 143: 285-6.

Lesson #100 is a surgical environmental law. It eliminates the pollution of drain discussions on our wards, in our operating theaters, surgical conferences and lounges.

By eliminating drain discussions at the Matrix Conference, we will contribute to the science and progress of surgery.

Epilogue

These are the Matrix Lessons.

These are the essential lessons of medical life; lessons not available in the standard texts. These lessons give you insight into this marvelous discipline we call clinical medicine. For surgical residents, these lessons are guideposts of enlightenment along the serpiginous trail of surgical education. For the medical practitioner, these lessons are insights into a complex profession. All lessons in medicine are the subject of continuing debate and reassessment. Some of my colleagues, particularly those of the professorial persuasion, may regard these lessons with some disdain.

One full-professor-in-waiting called these lessons a "ragtag collection of innuendo, rumor and half truth." But I would caution the skeptical reader:

- All rumors are true. I learned this from the motion picture "The Player."
- At least a half truth is half true. We just have to figure out the other half.
- The innuendo is the most logical, least risky and certainly the most entertaining method of transmitting knowledge in medicine.

If one perfects his innuendo techniques; if one makes the innuendo his hallmark; if one can captivate one's colleagues by this method, then one has a shot at becoming the master of the innuendo which, in surgical parlance, is also known as - the chief of surgery.

We now come to the end of this treatise. It began with a Ciceronian quote. Cicero tells us that there are lessons not found in books, but lessons we learn "which we have caught up from nature herself, sucked in and imbibed." As physicians, we have learned many lessons by this method:

- Lessons no professor ever taught us.
- Lessons no book could ever reveal to us.
- Lessons learned in the gray dawn of a New England morning, in the biting cold of a Chicago night and in the cool sunset of a California evening.
- Lessons bursting into our consciousness as we deal with distorted anatomy.
- Lessons forever imprinted on our minds as we sit with grieving families.
- Lessons we have learned as our careers and our lives have progressed.
- Lessons "... written on the fleshy tablets of the heart."